"Far too many people silently suffer with this disabling body,
Claiborn and Pedrick expertly offer the information and interventions to help individuals with body dysmorphic disorder create the needed balance in their body image experiences and their lives. *The BDD Workbook* is an excellent and essential resource for mental health professionals wishing to provide mindfully innovative therapeutic care."

—Thomas F. Cash, Ph.D., Professor of Psychology, Old Dominion University, author, *The Body Image Workbook*

"This book provides clear and practical guidelines that should be of considerable help to those many persons suffering from Body Dysmorphic Disorder. It should help to raise awareness about a problem that has not been widely recognized until recently."

—Edmund J. Bourne, Ph.D., author, *The Anxiety and Phobia Workbook*

"As I read *The BDD Workbook,* I kept wishing that such a wonderful resource had been available to me when I first started showing signs of Body Dysmorphic Disorder nearly thirty years ago. I found this book to be a thoughtful, step-by-step guide that will be extraordinarily valuable to BDD sufferers, their families, and to clinicians. I congratulate the authors for putting together this rich, easy-to-read manual, which clearly offers new hope to those of us living with BDD and related disorders."

—Scott M. Granet, L.C.S.W., Psychotherapist and President of the Obsessive-Compulsive Foundation of the San Francisco Bay Area

"*The BDD Workbook* is an impressive contribution to the small body of existing literature for people struggling with body image concerns and for mental health care professionals. Claiborn and Pedrick offer a thorough descriptive discussion of BDD as well as a practical, user-friendly presentation of cognitive-behavioral intervention strategies. Specifically, the numerous worksheets, exercises, and clinical examples allow both patients and practitioners to understand the utility of CBT for BDD. The authors maintain a compassionate and hopeful voice throughout this valuable resource."

—Barbara Van Noppen, M.S.W., Research Associate, Brown University Department of Psychiatry

"Claiborn and Pedrick have produced in *The BDD Workbook* a simple, straightforward aid for sufferers of body image concerns. In cases of mild discomfort or severe anguish the exercises in this book will be of great help to anyone experiencing the pain of BDD or body image problems. We at the Neysa Jane Body Dysmorphic Fund, Inc. are glad to see a new tool to help people with BDD get back to happy active lives."

—James W. Powley, President, Neysa Jane Body
Dysmorphic Fund, Inc.

THE BDD WORKBOOK

Overcome Body Dysmorphic Disorder
and End Body Image Obsessions

JAMES CLAIBORN, PH.D. & CHERRY PEDRICK, R.N.

NEW HARBINGER PUBLICATIONS, INC.

Publisher's Note

This publication is designed to provide accurate and authoritative information in regard to the subject matter covered. It is sold with the understanding that the publisher is not engaged in rendering psychological, financial, legal, or other professional services. If expert assistance or counseling is needed, the services of a competent professional should be sought.

Distributed in Canada by Raincoast Books

Copyright © 2002 by James Claiborn and Cherry Pedrick
New Harbinger Publications, Inc.
5674 Shattuck Avenue
Oakland, CA 94609

Cover design by Salmon Studios
Cover photo by Robert Farber/Corbis
Edited by Karen O'Donnell Stein
Text design by Tracy Carlson

ISBN-10 1-57224-293-0
ISBN-13 978-1-57224-293-7

Printed in the United States of America

New Harbinger Publications' website address: www.newharbinger.com

17   16   15

15   14   13   12   11   10   9   8

Contents

Part I
Understanding Body Dysmorphic Disorder

Part II
The Balanced Image Program

Acknowledgments

I started giving out advice and self-help tips on the Internet a number of years ago. That put me in contact with hundreds of people struggling with problems like obsessive-compulsive disorder and body dysmorphic disorder. I have learned an immense amount from them and hope I have given them some tools for managing their problems as well as hope for the future. I want to thank them for their patience with me as I learned. I also thank my wife Carolyn and my children, who have tolerated my long hours at the computer. Cherry Pedrick, my coauthor, has been inspiring and made this book possible.

—James M. Claiborn, Ph.D. ABPP

Writing has become a second career for me. Over the years, I've been encouraged, instructed, and mentored by people too numerous to mention. I would like to thank the writer's group that meets at the bookstore on Rainbow Boulevard every Wednesday. You all have been an inspiration to me. I am grateful for my online writer friends and supporters. You know who you are. I am thankful to my husband, Jim, and my son, James, for their support and encouragement, and to my coauthor, James Claiborn, who has been wonderful to work with. Most of all, I thank my God for making it all possible.

—Cherry Pedrick, R.N.

We would both like to thank Katharine A. Phillips, M.D., for allowing us to use the Body Dysmorphic Disorder Questionnaire (BDDQ). We also thank her and her colleagues, Eric Hollander, Steven Rasmussen, Bonnie Aronowitz, Concetta DeCaria, and Wayne Goodman, for the use of their Body Dysmorphic Disorder Modification of the Y-BOCS (BDD-YBOCS). We are also grateful to James C. Rosen, Ph.D., and Jeff Reifer, Ph.D., for allowing us to use the BDDE-SR. These researchers and others continue to work diligently for the benefit of those throughout the world who suffer with body dysmorphic disorder. We are thankful to Karen O'Donnell Stein, our editor, who helped us make *The BDD Workbook* more understandable and inviting and al the others at New Harbinger Publications who made this book a reality.

Introduction

D o you have a balanced body image? If not, it's possible that you fall into one of two groups: those who have body dysmorphic disorder (BDD), and those who are concerned about their body image but not so concerned that it greatly interferes with their life. To be diagnosed with BDD, a person's preoccupation with body image must cause significant distress or impairment of functioning. This disorder affects average-looking people who have great concerns about slight imperfections or imagined defects in their appearance. *The BDD Workbook* is a plan of action, a step-by-step program that people in both groups—those with BDD, and those who are overly concerned with their body image—can use to improve their lives. So what do we mean by *balanced body image*? Several components make up a balanced body image:

- **Balanced body-image perception.** Everybody has a perceived body image and an ideal body image. Your perceived body image is the mental picture you have of yourself. It may be quite realistic, much like the perception others have of you, or it may be slightly or greatly distorted. You may see your body as one sees his or her body in a trick mirror that distorts images. Or you may see just one part of your body in this distorted fashion. A balanced body-image perception is a realistic body image, similar to the view others have of you.

- **Balanced body-image response.** Every person responds in some way to his or her perceived body image. You may respond in positive ways, or in quite negative ways. We realize that by reading this book you may not change your perception of your body image. In fact, we won't try very hard to help you do this. But you can choose to *respond* differently to your perceived body image. We will help you examine your response to you perceived body image and make some positive changes in that response. A balanced response to your body image is one that allows you to accept your perceptions and limit the distress or interference with your life.

- **Balanced ideal body image.** Everybody also has an ideal body image. This is the body image you aspire to attain. Perhaps your ideal image is not realistic. It may be out of your reach; most of us can't look like the models we see on television and in magazines. A balanced ideal body image is one that is realistic or within reach.

- **Balanced ideal-body-image response.** Just as a person responds to a body image, he or she also responds to an ideal body image. We'll help you examine the images you see in the media and learn to make healthier, more constructive responses. A balanced ideal-body-image response is one that is accepting, realistic, and positive.

- **Balanced self-image.** Many people's self-esteem is wrapped up in how they look or how they think they look. You will learn alternative ways of defining yourself. When you put less emphasis on your body image and more emphasis on who you are, your self-esteem, and your self-image, will improve. A balanced self-image is one that includes body, mind, and spirit. It encompasses all the positive things about you, and the plans you have for positive, realistic change.

How This Book Can Help You

The BDD Workbook is not intended to be a substitute for treatment by a qualified mental health professional. Rather, it can be used in the following ways:

- As an adjunct to treatment with a professional. For example, you may be seeing a qualified mental health professional who does not specialize in the treatment of BDD. *The BDD Workbook* can assist your therapist in his or her role of coach, guide, and adviser as you work to bring your body image into balance.

- By helping people who are not in need of ongoing professional help. You may have a desire to learn as much about BDD as possible, using this book as a guide for self-directed intervention. If, while reading this book, you realize that you may have BDD, we urge you to see a mental health professional who is experienced in the diagnosis and treatment of BDD and the spectrum of related disorders. A psychiatrist or psychologist can confirm a diagnosis of BDD and help you decide whether self-directed cognitive behavioral therapy is appropriate for you. If you are depressed or have had thoughts of suicide (very common among people with BDD), it is imperative that you seek help immediately.

- By helping people who are dissatisfied with their body images, but whose concerns don't approach the severity of BDD. The same treatment principles apply to this milder form of body-image dissatisfaction. *The BDD Workbook* provides methods to reduce your dissatisfaction and distress.

- By assisting family members and mental health professionals who seek a better understanding of BDD and body image problems. *The BDD Workbook* can help them provide positive support to those struggling with BDD or body-image dissatisfaction.

Image Balancing Strategy

We all have a perceived body image and an ideal body image. One of the goals of the Balanced Image Program is to help you bring about a more satisfying balance between your perceived body image and your ideal body image. In what ways is your body image out of balance?

The BDD Workbook is divided into two parts. Part I will help you understand body dysmorphic disorder and related concerns. We will discuss the role of culture and how our response to images presented by the entertainment and advertising industries, and peer pressure, can affect body-image satisfaction. You will learn how BDD is diagnosed, what the symptoms are, and how the disorder is treated. We will help you assess your problem with body image. The Balanced Image Program involves change. You will learn about the process of change and decide whether you want to make important changes in the way you view your body.

Part II is the core of the book. We will give you step-by-step instructions guiding you through the Balanced Image Program. Throughout the book, but especially in these chapters, you will be asked to answer questions and complete charts. Doing so is important because each step builds on the last step. Information gathered in the first chapters will be used in subsequent chapters, so be prepared to put pen or pencil to paper and work the program, from start to finish. A more balanced self-image will be your reward. You'll learn to reach out to others as you struggle with body-image problems; family and friends can play important roles in your process of change.

The BDD Workbook will require your participation. Exercises and worksheets will help you collect information and understand your problem with body image. The goals of the Balanced Image Program are to help you narrow the gap between your perceived body image and your ideal body image, improve your response to your perceived body image and your ideal body image, and reduce the importance of body image in your overall self-image. The Image Balancing Strategies, like the one below, will remind you of key points in *The BDD Workbook* and help you stay focused on your efforts to bring about a more balanced self-image. Copy these strategies and tape them to your refrigerator door, keep them in your car or purse, or place them by your favorite chair.

From the Authors

Jim Claiborn, Ph.D.

I am a psychologist who is interested in how people can change their behavior. When my fellow students in school were fascinated by Freud, I was reading about Skinner and behavior modification. I have always been interested in behavioral and cognitive methods for changing behavior. Part of my fascination comes from the fact that these methods are both simple and effective. I earned a Ph.D. in Counseling Psychology in 1978 and have been in practice ever since. In the last several years I have focused much of my work on obsessive-compulsive disorder and related disorders. Body dysmorphic disorder is part of that group of related disorders. This book is designed to bring what I have learned over the years to people with body image problems including BDD and to try to ease their suffering.

Cherry Pedrick, R.N.

After twenty years working as a registered nurse, I made a career change. In 1995, I took up mouse and keyboard and pursued a writing career. I wrote articles for several magazines, then coauthored *The OCD Workbook* with Bruce M. Hyman, Ph.D., in 1999. I coauthored *The Habit Change Workbook* with Dr. Claiborn in 2001. We had such a good time working together that we teamed up again to write *The BDD Workbook*. My interest in cognitive behavioral therapy began when I used its principles in the treatment of my own obsessive-compulsive disorder (OCD). As you will see, OCD and BDD are related in some ways and the treatments are similar.

PART I

Understanding Body Dysmorphic Disorder

Chapter 1

What Is Body Dysmorphic Disorder?

The *Diagnostic and Statistical Manual of Mental Disorders*, fourth edition (*DSM-IV-TR*) (APA 2000), which provides a diagnostic system for mental health, describes BDD as a preoccupation with a defect in appearance. The defect is either imagined or minor. If a defect is present, the individual's concern about the defect is markedly excessive in comparison with the severity of the defect. This preoccupation causes significant distress or impairment in social, occupational, or other areas of functioning. The preoccupation is not better accounted for by another disorder, such as anorexia nervosa; in other words, it is not the result of or part of another disorder.

A Closer Look

Put more simply, body dysmorphic disorder is diagnosed when a person is excessively preoccupied or focused on some defect or problem in his or her appearance. You will meet a few people with BDD later, and you will learn that the preoccupation can concern any body part. Later in this book you will read about Cameron, who thinks his nose is too long and bumpy; Lilly, who thinks her thighs are misshapen and repulsive; and Arnold, who thinks his cheeks are too red and make him look childish. These people are not just a little uncomfortable; they are obsessed with their appearance problems. Thoughts about their defects intrude into their minds and cause them great suffering.

Studies have found that almost everyone is at times unhappy with some aspect of his or her appearance (Cash 1997). Who hasn't looked in the mirror and thought, "I wish I were thinner," or looked at the snapshots of a Christmas party and thought, "Gee, I'm really getting bald"? For those of us who don't have BDD, these thoughts are passing ones. When we are confronted with those flaws we may feel a little uncomfortable or try to make an adjustment to improve our looks, but then we move on to other thoughts. People who have BDD just can't move on. The thoughts get stuck and cause great distress.

The *DSM-IV-TR* refers to the defect as either imagined or slight. But, clearly, to people with BDD the defects are present and are not slight. When they tell others about their concern, which they are often reluctant to do, other people will usually say, "I don't know what you are talking about," "I don't see it," or "It's not a problem." The person with BDD believes that the speaker is just being polite—"They're just being nice; they don't want to hurt my feelings." Dr. Claiborn has had many patients sit in his office describing their defects and, even when looking closely, he usually can't see them at all. If he tells patients that he doesn't see the flaw, their usual reaction is to tell him that he is just being a proper professional and trying to make them feel better. The *DSM-IV-TR*'s description of the defect as imagined or slight refers to the judgment of others, not of the individual with BDD. To the person with BDD, the defect is usually both quite real and severe.

The *DSM-IV-TR* also describes the reaction to the defect as excessive. Again, this description refers to an outsider's judgment. The individual with the problem may not see their reaction as excessive at all. He or she might say, "If you had a horrible deformity you would be upset too!" The individual's perception of the importance and realness of the defect is what mental health professionals call *insight*. In working with people with BDD, we see a range of levels of insight, from people who know their defect is really minor to people who view it as catastrophic.

To better understand the concept of insight, let's look at insight in people with phobias. Suppose you had a fear of spiders. If the fear were limiting your life we would probably tell you that you had a spider phobia, or an irrational fear of spiders. Most people with this type of problem have enough insight into the fear be able to say, "I know my fear is out of proportion, but I can't help it." Recognition of the distorted or exaggerated reaction is also insight. It is common for people with BDD to have little or no insight into the degree of exaggeration of their response. This presents some challenge for treatment, because if the individual sees his or her concern as justified then he or she would have little reason to seek help from a mental health professional. Since the defect is seen as real and important, it makes much more sense to him or her to go to a dermatologist or a plastic surgeon. Later in this chapter we will talk about this issue again.

The definition of BDD includes significant distress or impairment of function on the part of the sufferer, which can take many forms. One of the most common forms of impairment is serious depression, or *clinical depression*. Researchers have found that serious depression occurs in over 80 percent of patients seeking treatment for BDD, at some point during their lives (Phillips 1999). Depression is often accompanied by suicidal thoughts and attempts, but even people who have BDD without severe depression may have thoughts of suicide. Dr. Katharine Phillips, an expert on BDD, reports that 86 percent of her patients with BDD have had thoughts of suicide—thoughts that life wasn't worth living or that they would be better off dead because of their despair about their appearance problem. About 25 percent of Dr. Phillips' patients with BDD have actually attempted suicide, and most related the reason to their appearance concerns (Phillips 1996).

In addition to being associated with depression and suicidal thoughts, BDD interferes with functioning in other ways. People with body-image problems such as BDD may spend large amounts of time and money trying to correct their perceived defects. They can get into financial difficulty or drastically limit other activities as a result. Often, they avoid situations in which they fear others will see their defect, sometimes to the point of being diagnosed with social phobia. In fact, many people with BDD also meet the criteria for a diagnosis of social phobia. Like depression, social phobia may be a co-morbid disorder, a disorder that coexists with another, such as BDD, and influences how the BDD affects the individual's life. While the individual may have social phobia in addition to BDD, the person making the diagnosis may miss the BDD, seeing only the avoidance and fear associated with social situations and treating only the social phobia. This treatment will usually not be effective since it does not address the BDD that drives the social avoidance. Whether they meet the criteria for social phobia or not, most people with BDD will avoid some situations or take special precautions when they are out in public to deal with their appearance concerns.

How Common Is Body Dysmorphic Disorder?

Body dysmorphic disorder is more common than was previously thought. Although the disorder was described clearly in the 1880s (Phillips 1996) it was considered rare until recently. Only a small number of articles were written about the disorder. Early descriptions used the term *dysmorphophobia*. (The use of the root *phobia* implies an irrational fear, which does not match the modern description of BDD.) The diagnostic term *body dysmorphic disorder* became official when it appeared in the 1987 publication of the *DSM-III-R*

(APA 1987). Since then, a small number of researchers have become interested in BDD, and our understanding of it has grown rapidly. Unlike with many better-studied and more well-known disorders, we still don't have enough solid research to tell us how common BDD is, but it is estimated to occur in 1 to 2 percent of the general population. BDD may be found in 4 to 5 percent of people seeking medical treatment, in 8 percent of people with depression, and in up to 12 percent of people seeking outpatient mental health treatment (Phillips 1996).

Not enough data exists to show whether this disorder is equally common in men and women, but clinical experience seems to suggest that it is. There appear to be more concerns over muscles and hair loss in males, and perhaps more focus on skin appearance and breast, leg, or buttock size or shape in women. However, any of these concerns can show up in either gender. It is quite common for people with BDD to have more than one "defect" that they are upset about.

BDD Symptoms

What exactly are the symptoms of BDD? Two major features make up BDD: the preoccupation with the defect, and the actions people take to reduce their feelings of distress. The person with BDD spends a lot of time thinking about the defect and worrying about how others will react or what they will think. When assessing the severity of BDD, mental health professionals consider the amount of time spent thinking about or being preoccupied with these concerns. Most of us spend only a few minutes each day thinking about our appearance, but the typical person with BDD may spend hours worrying about how he or she looks.

The other major feature of this disorder is what people do to reduce their distress. We have already discussed how this distress can be so severe that it leads to depression, suicide, and avoidance of other people or situations where others may see the defect. Appearance concerns can also lead the person to spend large amounts of time trying to check, assess, or fix the problem. These actions can take the form of measuring, weighing, and looking in the mirror. Some people with BDD spend long hours looking at themselves to see if the defect is noticeable or has changed in some way. They may pose in front of the mirror or try to act a certain way in public to make the defect hidden or at least less noticeable. Others spend hours applying makeup, changing clothes, or rearranging hair in order to correct or cover up the problem. Others with BDD spend hours picking at their skin in an effort to remove imperfections or make the skin surface even. Although it may seem contradictory, people who are preoccupied with defects in their body may often develop a habit of picking at their skin. Although often described as an attempt to fix a blemish or remove an imperfection, this behavior can result in scars, wounds that are never allowed to heal, and in rare cases even life-threatening health problems. To someone without BDD, picking seems especially self-defeating in an individual who is obsessed with imperfections in their skin. This is only one of the ironies of the disorder. In addition, people with this disorder will often repeatedly seek reassurance from others that the problem is not terribly obvious or that it has been adequately disguised.

Some people with BDD are so uncomfortable showing themselves in public that they become housebound. This behavior can be mistaken for agoraphobia. Agoraphobia is defined in the *DSM-IV-TR* (APA 2000) as anxiety about being in places from which escape might be difficult or embarrassing, or places in which help might not be available. Agoraphobia can lead a person to avoid crossing bridges or going to public places, or even leaving the house. Although the external behavior may seem similar, BDD differs from agoraphobia in that the avoidance of public place stems from embarrassment about appearance rather than fear of becoming trapped or stranded.

Researchers have compiled statistics about the body parts people with BDD focus on. The face is the most common body part that people with BDD worry about. The concern can be about some specific part of the face, such as the nose, lips, or ears, or it can include facial skin appearance, including wrinkles, color, blemishes, scars, veins, texture, or pore size. Hair and hairlines are also commonly the focus of concern. The focus of attention can be any body feature, frequently the size or shape of legs, arms, buttocks, breasts, or genitals. While people with eating disorders such as anorexia nervosa are usually very concerned with general body weight or being fat, people with BDD focus on specific parts of the body.

One form of BDD is known as *muscle dysmorphia*, or what one group of authors call the "Adonis Complex" in their ground-breaking book, *The Adonis Complex: The Secret Crisis of Male Body Obsession* (Pope, Phillips, and Olivardia 2000). This problem is seen primarily in men, who usually perceive themselves as puny, or not muscular enough. Thus, like others with BDD, they see parts of their body as defective. They often spend hours engaged in extreme exercise regimes, wear clothing that hides their bodies, and avoid going places, such as the beach, where they would be expected to take off their shirts. Some eat special diets or even use drugs such as anabolic steroids to try to correct the perceived problem.

What Causes BDD?

The short answer is that we don't know the cause of BDD. Theories exist but much more research is needed before we will have a good answer to this question. If we look at average individuals, we find that most people have dissatisfaction with some aspect of their appearance at some point in their lives. There is evidence showing that body-image dissatisfaction has actually become a more common problem in recent years. A survey in 1972, in which people were asked questions about body-image dissatisfaction, found that 36 percent of men and 50 percent of women reported dissatisfaction with their mid-torso. In a 1996 survey, the rate of dissatisfaction was found to have risen to 63 percent of men and 71 percent of women. Similarly, discontent about overall appearance went from 15 percent to 43 percent in men and 23 percent to 56 percent in women in the same time period (Cash 1997). Of course, these people did not *all* have BDD, and ordinary body-image concern does not lead to the development of BDD. The problem is more complex than that, but the results do make it clear that things are happening in our world that lead to body-image concerns in a large number of people.

Despite the increase of body-image dissatisfaction in the general population, something different seems to be going on in people who develop BDD. Is the cause some childhood trauma, possible child abuse or excessive teasing? There is no evidence that a history of abuse is any more common in people who develop BDD. Interestingly, while many people with BDD recount how they were teased about some aspect of their appearance, that body part may not be the same one that preoccupies them now. In addition, the type of teasing they describe, or the critical event that some identify as the beginning of their BDD, is often no different from the experiences of people without BDD. Almost everybody has been teased about appearance at some point in their lives, and many may be the victims of prolonged, cruel treatment by peers or even family. However, most people don't develop BDD. Later we will tell you about two people: Jamila, who during childhood was teased about her long fingers, and Cameron, who was teased about his nose. Did this cause them to have BDD? We don't think so. Other factors are likely to have predisposed them to BDD, although the teasing may have influenced what body parts concerned them the most or contributed to developing the problem.

Some experts argue that BDD is a genetic disorder. At this point, the data is too limited for us to be able to determine the importance of genetic factors, although, as with other disorders such as obsessive-compulsive disorder, the possibility of some sort of genetic predisposition seems reasonable. Is BDD caused by our culture's emphasis on appearance and our concepts of beauty? We are certainly bombarded with messages telling us what looks good, what makes people attractive, and that whatever we look like now is not good enough. We are told we can't be happy or loved unless our hair is the right color, we are slim and fit, and we smell good. However, we know that BDD has been around for years, even before these messages began their assault. We are all influenced by the content of these messages, and they may even contribute to an increase in the incidence of BDD, but if these messages were the cause of BDD we would expect almost everyone to have the disorder.

We will discuss some disorders that appear related to BDD next. Theories about what causes them may apply to BDD as well.

Related Disorders

When scientists look at research findings and try to understand them, they look for patterns. When we study disorders like BDD we sometimes think in patterns and related disorders. One model includes the idea that BDD is one of a spectrum of depressive disorders. A point in favor of this argument are the facts that depression occurs in such a high percentage of people with BDD and, conversely, that so many people with depression have major concerns about their appearance. There is also a high rate of depression in the families of people who develop BDD. Another point in support of this model is that a group of antidepressant medications seem to work reasonably well as a treatment for BDD. These antidepressants work by changing the way the brain handles serotonin, a chemical messenger or neurotransmitter. On the other hand, many antidepressants that affect other brain chemicals don't seem to help BDD, although they work for many people with depression.

The other spectrum model takes into account the similarities between BDD and obsessive-compulsive disorder (OCD). Like people with OCD, people with BDD have obsessions. In OCD the obsessions can be about almost any topic, such as harming others or contamination. People with BDD have obsessions, but the obsessions are focused on their own appearance. People with OCD engage in rituals or compulsions, such as checking to make sure certain things are all right, excessive washing, and avoiding situations that might trigger obsessions. People with BDD often engage in repeated checking of their appearance and avoid situations where they would be exposed to triggers for their concerns. Both disorders respond to the same treatments, with cognitive behavioral therapy and antidepressants that affect serotonin, although BDD may be more difficult to treat than OCD. Approximately 80 to 90 percent of people with BDD have problems with depression, while only about 30 percent seem to have OCD.

The skin-picking problem we mentioned earlier turns out to be common in people with OCD and in people with trichotillomania (compulsive hair pulling), as well as in those with BDD. Trichotillomania often overlaps with both OCD and BDD, supporting the idea that the three disorders are part of a common spectrum. Most people with OCD have insight about the exaggerated response that is part of their disorder, at least some of the time. In BDD, it is common for people to have little or no insight into their exaggerated response and to be firmly convinced that their defect is not only real, but also significant and noticeable. Sometimes this belief is so strong that it is described as a delusion. A delusion is a false belief that is held despite the fact that almost everyone else doesn't accept it and despite a complete lack of evidence supporting it and even lots of evidence refuting it. Delusions are usually thought of as part of psychotic disorders such as schizophrenia. However, delusions seen in schizophrenia are often bizarre and treatments that work for schizophrenia don't seem useful for BDD, making a relationship between these two disorders seem unlikely.

Special attention needs to be paid to the question of a relationship between BDD and eating disorders such as anorexia nervosa. The *DSM-IV-TR* (APA 2000) says specifically that when anorexia is diagnosed, BDD should not also be diagnosed unless the excessive preoccupation is unrelated to excess weight. But despite the different diagnostic labels, there are many similarities. Like those with BDD, people with anorexia are preoccupied with and very distressed about their appearance. They may go to great efforts to try to correct their appearance, including dressing in clothes to hide their "fat" and avoiding situations where their bodies can be viewed. People with eating disorders spend much of their time dealing with eating and food. They may have rituals that they feel they must perform in order to make eating permissible or to rid themselves of unwanted weight. Like people with BDD, they seem caught up in an exaggerated sense of the importance of body image. One study (Jolanta and Tomasz 2000) found that 25 percent of women diagnosed with anorexia showed clear evidence of BDD symptoms before the anorexia was present. (Unlike BDD, anorexia is predominantly found in women. As we indicated earlier, BDD seems to be a much more equal-opportunity disorder, occurring at about the same rate in males and females. Some authors have described muscle dysmorphia, which occurs more often in males, as "reverse anorexia" and in some ways this is an apt description.)

If you have an eating disorder like anorexia nervosa you may find it helpful to use this workbook and its exercises to help you with your body-image distress. Since anorexia is a life-threatening disorder we strongly urge you to get professional help for it. You can show this book to your therapist, who may want to make some adjustments in how you use it.

BDD and Health-Care Professionals

If most people who have BDD don't recognize that they have exaggerated concerns, then they are unlikely to go to a mental health professional for help. After all, if you are upset about your appearance you aren't likely to go to someone to talk about feelings—you are probably going to look for help with your appearance problem. People who have concerns about the shape of their nose or other facial features, for example, may consult a plastic surgeon. If the surgeon says the problem is not worth fixing, the person with BDD is likely to move on to another doctor. The surgeon may agree that the defect is minor but changeable, but this doesn't provide a satisfactory answer either: often, the individual will be satisfied with the results of surgery at first, only to become obsessed with the same body part again. The individual may even think the surgery was botched and made the defect worse. Tragically, they may seek repeated surgery, take legal action, or even try to get revenge against the surgeon for ruining their appearance. There are some reports of people with BDD being happy with the results of surgery, but as far as we can tell this is an exception rather than a rule.

The health-care providers who may see the largest number of people with BDD are dermatologists. This makes sense since many people with BDD have skin or hair concerns and skin picking is common. It seems only logical that if you thought you had a defect or problem with your skin you would go to a skin doctor. In a large case series of people seen in a psychiatric setting for BDD, 46 percent had sought treatment from a dermatologist and 38 percent had received treatment from one. Like people with BDD who seek plastic surgery, most patients were not satisfied with the treatment from the dermatologist and only 13 percent thought the problem had improved (Phillips, et al. 2000)

In the 2000 study by Phillips and her colleagues almost 12 percent of the people who had seen dermatologists were found to have BDD and over 15 percent of those with minimal or nonexistent defects had BDD. Most of the patients reported severe or extreme distress or interference with daily functioning as a result of the perceived defect. Body dysmorphic disorder patients often end up going from one dermatologist to another when they are unsatisfied with the results of treatment, or they may insist on treatments that are not needed or won't help. They may ask for frequent reassurance from the doctor, but this reassurance doesn't seem to make them feel better, or at least not for long. If there is a real defect or skin problem, or if the skin is damaged from picking, treatment by the dermatologist may help, but is unlikely to be enough by itself. What is needed is a change in the individual's excessive body-image concern.

The Disgust Problem

We have discussed how OCD, trichotillomania, and depression might be related to BDD. However, the *DSM-IV-TR* defines depression as a mood disorder and OCD as an anxiety disorder. Trichotillomania is called an impulse control disorder and BDD a somatoform disorder. These disorders are classified according to their complaints. Somatoform disorders, including BDD, generally involve concerns with aspects of the body or its function. For example, people with hypochondriasis, another somatoform disorder, are convinced they are ill, despite the fact that there is no objective evidence to support their belief. This belief is not very different from the conviction that there is something wrong with the appearance of the body when there isn't.

The biggest difference is in the emotional reaction to the perceived problem. Most people with hypochondriasis have such tremendous anxiety that some experts refer to the disorder as "health anxiety," and most people with OCD and other anxiety disorders have significant anxiety about some sort of perceived danger. People with BDD, however, seem more disgusted and ashamed of their appearance than they do anxious. Disgust shows up in some anxiety disorders such as OCD and phobias, and recently some researchers have paid special attention to it. At this point, however, disgust is less understood scientifically than anxiety is. Understanding disgust is a critical part of developing a treatment for BDD and related body-image problems. In chapter 9 we will look at how you can work with disgust, which will be somewhat different from the approach we would use to treat anxiety problems. An important goal in working with body-image problems is to get to the point where you are no longer disgusted by your own body. This is not the same as believing your body is perfect, which is not a reasonable goal. It is about accepting who you are and how you look.

You Are Not Alone

It helps to know that you aren't alone in your struggle with body-image dissatisfaction. The people you will meet here are representatives of the millions of people who are dissatisfied with their bodies. Some have diagnosable body dysmorphic disorder (BDD) and may have other conditions that can complicate BDD, such as obsessive-compulsive disorder, depression, trichotillomania, social phobia, or agoraphobia. We have also included descriptions of people who have body-image dissatisfaction that isn't severe enough to be diagnosed as BDD; while this dissatisfaction isn't as devastating as BDD, it can still cause distress and interfere with a person's ability to lead a fulfilling life. These are composites of patients with BDD; you may find similarities between yourself and one or more of the people described, but this is only coincidental. We'll follow these people throughout the book.

Arnold's Story

After several sessions with his therapist, whom he was seeing for depression, Arnold revealed the problems that were bothering him the most. He thought his eyes were too small and his cheeks too red, and he felt that this made him appear childish and weak. He usually wore sunglasses to hide his eyes and avoided the sun and exercise because these might have made his cheeks even rosier. Arnold, fearing rejection because of his "weak and childish" appearance, was underemployed and lacked the confidence to get a good job. He frequently questioned his friends and family about his cheeks and eyes, and they all reassured him that they looked fine.

Morgan's Story

Years ago, Morgan had picked at a pimple on her chin. Though no one else could see it, she insisted there was a scar. She was also embarrassed about the dark circles under her eyes; they seemed darker and much deeper to her than to anyone else. When she was tired, the dark circles seemed worse. Morgan had applied numerous brands of skin lightening creams to the "scar" on her chin and eye creams and gels to the skin around her eyes. She was usually happy with the results for a day or two, but then the dissatisfaction would return and she'd search for new treatments. She spent hours checking her face in mirrors and poring over skin-care articles in beauty magazines. Afraid that people would stare at her face, Morgan lived with her parents and almost never left the house.

Alfred's Story

To hide his arms, Alfred usually wore long sleeved shirts, even at the gym. He worked out everyday, trying to get his arms to "look right." To him, they were hideously misshapen and much too small. When he did have to wear a short-sleeved shirt, Alfred would hold his arms close to his sides or folded in front of him. Still, he didn't feel right, so he tried to avoid situations where his arms would be exposed. More and more, he stayed home, because he began to feel that even his wrists looked deformed. Eventually he stopped going out at all. Alfred weighed himself several times a day and ate large amounts to keep up his weight, convinced that the extra pounds would make his arms larger and more "normal." He spent at least an hour a day in front of the mirror, trying out different arm positions to make them look better. Alfred compared his arms to those of models in bodybuilding magazines and felt that his life would be fine if only he could get his arms looking right.

Lilly's Story

Lilly tried diets, exercise, and creams, but nothing seemed to make her stomach and thighs look right to her. She wore loose clothing and wouldn't go swimming or wear shorts. When the family went to the beach she wore long, loose sundresses that camouflaged what she described as "grotesque thighs" and "a fat, repulsive stomach." Dressing and bathing were ordeals for her because she would get "stuck" in front of the mirror, examining her stomach and thighs. Lilly compared herself with models in magazines and on TV, paying special attention to their stomachs and thighs. Her husband insisted she had a beautiful figure, but in fact he worried that she was getting too thin.

Duncan's Story

As a teenager, Duncan had acne. He picked at the blemishes, trying to smooth the rough spots. When he became an adult his acne cleared up, but he continued to worry about his skin. He was careful not to get scrapes or cuts, but when he did he picked at the sores, again trying to smooth his skin. He used the latest products to moisturize his skin and prevent the appearance of aging and sun damage. Still, Duncan felt that the skin on his forehead and cheeks was rough and flaky and had a brownish tinge. He went to a dermatologist, who could not see the flaky skin and saw no abnormalities or discoloration. The dermatologist referred him to a psychologist because of Duncan's extreme distress, anxiety, and depression.

Jamila's Story

As a child, Jamila's brother called her "Needle Hands" and teased her about her long fingers and big hands. The children in the neighborhood thought this was funny and teased her too. She ignored any kind words she received from adults praising her beauty and grace and concentrated on the teasing about her hands. When she was being teased Jamila would smile and not let on that the nickname bothered her. When she got older, she went to college but dropped out after the first year. She felt quite sure that her classmates were offended by her large hands and turned their faces away in disgust. She moved back home with her parents and rarely went out. They worried about her and tried to get her involved in activities, but she refused, feeling too ashamed to tell them why she wouldn't go out.

Leo's Story

For Leo, everything had to be in order; he even alphabetized the foods in his kitchen cupboards. But most distressing was his hair, which he needed to always lie smoothly and evenly. Leo carried a small mirror in his pocket and checked his hair frequently. One side always seemed to stick out more than the other. After getting his hair cut, Leo would spend hours checking in the mirror to make certain his sideburns were even and the hairs were the same length on each side. Leo was shy around women. Not only did he obsess about his hair, but he also criticized himself for what he thought was vanity. Surely others would also think he was vain, he thought. Leo went to a therapist, who diagnosed and started treatment for obsessive-compulsive disorder. After several weeks, he revealed his appearance fears to his therapist, who diagnosed body dysmorphic disorder.

Delia's Story

Certain her hair was uneven, Delia, like Leo, dreaded getting haircuts. For days afterward, she would obsess about her hair. She would trim one side, then the other, spending hours measuring, obsessing, and trimming. Sometimes she pulled hairs that just didn't lie right or made her hairline uneven. Delia also obsessed about her eyebrows, plucking them to get them even, overdoing it, and then trying to let them grow again. Eyelashes were a problem too. They just didn't look right to her; some lashes didn't line up, so she would pull one lash. Then they were uneven so she would pull more hairs. As a result, her eyelashes were sometimes very thin, so she wore false eyelashes. She spent an hour on her makeup each day, paying special attention to her eyes. Skin blemishes also bothered Delia. She wanted her skin to be smooth and picked at any sores, scratches, or pimples. Delia went to a therapist, who diagnosed her with trichotillomania, in addition to body dysmorphic disorder.

Cameron's Story

In grade school, someone had called Cameron "Nosey." As he grew up he retained his self-consciousness about his nose. When people whispered at work, or even on the street, he thought they were talking about his long, bumpy nose and calling him names. Never happy with his nose, Cameron saved up to have plastic surgery. After having surgery on his nose, he was happy with it for several weeks. Then he decided it was still too long and looked "bumpy." He believed his coworkers were laughing at him. He felt that if even surgery couldn't make his nose look right, there was no hope.

Cameron consulted a second plastic surgeon to have his nose redone. During their consultation, Cameron revealed that he had also had extensive work done on his jaw by another plastic surgeon because he thought that one side was much larger than the other one. Since there actually was a slight asymmetry, the first doctor had done the surgery, but Cameron had been unhappy with the results. After two more surgeries, he resigned himself to having a "deformed" jaw. He mentioned that he had often considered suicide since he thought his face was hopelessly deformed. Upon hearing Cameron's story, the plastic surgeon referred him to a psychiatrist for consultation.

Casey's Story

At first, Casey was happy with her breasts after surgery. They were larger and fuller and she felt more confident and attractive. But then she became convinced that they were misshapen. Her husband insisted they looked fine. She examined her breasts in the mirror daily and insisted they were greatly distorted. Casey wore baggy clothes in an attempt to hide her breasts.

Paul's Story

Paul had gained a few pounds and joined a gym to get into shape. He worked out daily and lost the weight. Everyone said he looked great, but no matter how much he worked out he never looked as muscular as some of the guys at the gym. He quit his job at the bank and went to work at the gym, giving himself more time to work out. Paul took nutritional supplements offered for sale at the gym and changed his diet, which helped somewhat, but not enough for Paul. He got to know some of the other bodybuilders and learned their secret: they took anabolic steroids, purchased on the black market. After taking steroids for a while, Paul looked more like his bodybuilder friends. When he stopped taking them, he felt depressed and was convinced that the effects on his muscles diminished, so he started back on steroids.

Meanwhile, Paul's behavior become more aggressive. He totaled his car in an accident. Still, he drove recklessly and received several speeding tickets. He got in a fight with his neighbor and another with his brother. When he hit his wife, giving her a black eye, she gave him an ultimatum: Get help or she'd leave. Paul had been mild-mannered and easy to get along with until the last two years. He didn't see a connection between the aggression and the steroid use until he and his wife went to a marriage counselor, who explained that aggressive behavior and depression are very common side effects of anabolic steroid use.

Not Quite BDD

You may have body-image dissatisfaction that is not severe enough to fit the diagnosis of BDD. Perhaps you have experienced some of the BDD symptoms described in the stories above, but they have not significantly interfered with your life. Read on. You may find that they have more effect on your life than you think. Even if your symptoms are not severe enough to warrant a diagnosis of BDD, you can benefit from the same cognitive behavioral therapy principles used to help people with full-blown BDD. You may relate better to the people described below.

Linda's Story

Like many teenagers, Linda had moderate acne. She squeezed and picked at the pimples most evenings, then applied acne creams. Linda was also concerned about her hair. She wanted her long blond hair to always look nice. Linda was dissatisfied with her body image and felt she put too much emphasis on her appearance.

Calvin's Story

After spending thousands of dollars on hair products, Calvin was still losing hair. His hairline was slowly receding and he was developing a bald spot on the back of his head. Calvin was a successful businessman, but he felt his lack of hair was holding him back. His worries about hair loss were taking up more of his money and time than he would have liked.

Allison's Story

Though not overweight, Allison was on the upper end of the ideal weight tables for her height. Her body build was much like that of her mother, her sister, and most of the women in her family, but she wanted to be thin. Allison watched what she ate and exercised every day, attending group exercise classes and working out alone. She weighed herself daily and compared herself with her friends and models. She knew she could never be as thin as a model, but she wanted to be thinner than she was. Some of her classmates made themselves vomit after meals, took diet pills, exercised to excess, and smoked to maintain thin bodies. She was considering these options to control her weight.

Brad's Story

Although he was complimented for his body build, Brad was still unsatisfied. He went to the gym daily, ate a balanced diet, and took nutritional supplements. He was considering taking anabolic steroids despite the health risks. Brad debated whether looking like the men in the bodybuilding magazines would make taking the risks worthwhile.

Your Story

What about you? Now, on the page provided, briefly describe your struggle with body image. Later, you will more thoroughly examine your problem with body image.

 Image Balancing Strategy

It is important for your success that you answer all of the questions in the worksheets in this book as completely and honestly as possible.

To sum up, BDD is a very common disorder that is often missed by health-care providers. Mental health professionals usually recognize depression but often don't ask about BDD symptoms. Other health-care providers such as plastic surgeons, dermatologists, and primary-care physicians may not recognize depression and are even less likely than mental health professionals to ask about BDD. The majority of people with BDD never get proper treatment. Even if a person struggling with body-image issues goes to a mental health professional and brings up the possibility of BDD, he or she may not receive the necessary treatment, because the professional may not be aware of the best methods for treating the disorder.

Learning about BDD is just the beginning of your path to a more balanced self-image. After describing your body-image problem on the following page, go on to chapter 2. We will discuss the influence of today's culture on body-image dissatisfaction.

Your Body-Image Dissatisfaction Story

Write the story of your struggle with body-image dissatisfaction, describing the progression of your symptoms, from their inception to the present:

_____

_____

_____

_____

_____

_____

_____

_____

_____

_____

_____

_____

_____

_____

_____

_____

_____

Chart 1a

Lilly's Body-Image Dissatisfaction Story

Write the story of your struggle with body-image dissatisfaction, describing the progression of your symptoms, from their inception to the present:

Around the time that I turned thirteen, I noticed my stomach and thighs were large. They seemed to be much larger than those of my classmates. My brother teased me, calling me "Thunder Thighs." I know now he was just joking around, but at the time I thought that he was describing my thighs the way they really were. I began to wear loose clothing so no one could see just how fat my thighs were. I was embarrassed about my stomach too, which also seemed fat. As I left high school and entered college, I started to feel less embarrassed and disgusted with myself. I told myself I would just have to live with my looks. Then I got married and had two children. I gained weight after each child, only about ten pounds each, but it seemed to all go to my stomach and thighs. I was determined to get rid of the extra pounds and did lose weight, but my thighs and stomach looked as bad as ever. They are huge, grotesque, and repulsive. I've tried diets, exercise, and creams, but nothing seems to help. My husband says I look fine and worries that I've lost too much weight, but I think he's just saying that to be nice. I've got to either make myself look decent or accept myself the way I am. I don't feel I can do either. I hate bathing because I get stuck looking in the mirror at my thighs and stomach. I hate getting dressed because I can't find clothes that make me look right. I pore over magazines, looking for the secrets to looking decent, but then I get disgusted seeing all the beautiful models.

_____

_____

_____

_____

Chart 1b

CHAPTER 2

Cultural Influence on Body Image

Our culture has a great deal of influence on our body image. We view our bodies through a lens colored by the messages we receive from the media, the voice of the culture we live in. We don't always see our bodies realistically; even when we do, most of us find it impossible to live up to the ideal body image presented to us. In order to help get a more balanced understanding of this cultural influence, let's look briefly at the changes the ideal body has undergone throughout history.

Beauty Through the Ages

The definition of the ideal body has changed over the years, and it also differs from one culture to another. Body size and shape have always been seen as a sign of wealth and social status. When resources were scarce, a full figure was stylish because it indicated the ability to eat well. Larger bodies were also desired because they demonstrated probable health and fertility. Even in the Stone Age sculptors created round, voluptuous female sculptures with enormous stomachs. Between 1400 and 1700 a plump, big-breasted, maternal shape was fashionable. In the fifteenth century, following the bubonic plague, increasing the population was especially important. Women endeavored to look pregnant, with some even wearing pillows or stuffing under their dresses.

In the 1800s, the voluptuous female body was still popular, but now women wore corsets to tighten the waist and create an hourglass figure. Mid-century, the ideal body had large breasts, hips, and legs. Thinness was associated with illnesses, such as tuberculosis. In the United States the opulent 1920s saw the thin ideal for the first time, with the flat-chested, curveless flapper look. Suddenly, being thin showed you had *arrived*, distinguishing upper-class women from the poor immigrants coming to America. Some women even had plastic surgery to reduce the size of their breasts to achieve the look (today, women are more likely to have them enlarged). We saw narrow waists in the 1930s, slinky legs with high heels and garters in the 1940s, and large breasts in the 1950s and 1960s. The 1970s saw the beginning of the really thin ideal.

As you can see, the ideal body image of today is not the same as it was even as recently as the 1960s. Marilyn Monroe was five feet five inches tall and weighed up to 135 pounds at times. By today's standards for actresses and models, she would be considered overweight. Even the flapper girls of the 1920s wouldn't qualify as thin. The first Miss America (1922–23), Mary Campbell was a flapper and considered thin for that era; she was five feet seven inches and 140 pounds. Fashion models weighed 155 pounds and more. The thin bodies shown on TV, in movies, and in magazines today are relatively new.

How did the thin body image start? The diet, fashion, advertising, and entertainment industries have each made contributions to the development of the thin ideal. Dieting had its beginnings in the middle of the nineteenth century. At first, the aim was good health, but over time thinness became an ideal to strive for. Before the 1920s, people made their own clothing without the aid of preprinted sewing patterns. Ready-to-wear clothes and sewing patterns brought standard sizing and, with them, more emphasis on shape, dimension, and weight as people struggled to fit into standard sizes. Modern advertising, photography, and movies ushered in the fashion industry, which chose thinner frames to display fashions, partly to make up for the camera's distortion. Personal decisions about clothes and appearance became more influenced by outside forces. Today, designers are creating more plus-size clothing lines, but as a society we still have a long way to go before we can begin to celebrate the many shapes and sizes the human body can take.

In general, we've discussed female shapes, but men have been pressured to conform to certain sizes and shapes too, and stress for men in general is increasing. The uncertainties of today's world, with technological change, corporate downsizing, and increasing competition, have led men to feel more insecure and anxious. The right clothing, hair care, exercise, or diet may seem to be just the thing to increase a man's confidence and his belief that he will be more successful. We'll discuss this more in the next chapter.

Beauty Today

In the past, beauty ideals expressed through art were romanticized and not expected to be attainable. Today, photographic editing, soft-focus photography techniques, and airbrushing have blurred the line between fantasy and reality, making the ideals *seem* more attainable. A depiction of a model can even be made up of the features of several models: the face of one, the body of another, and the hair of yet another. In addition, the models and actresses look the way they do because of makeup, designer clothes, special diets, and exercise with the help of personal trainers. Deep down, most of us know that this is true, and we don't want to spend that much time on our looks, but we may feel that we should look just like a supermodel anyway.

Today, thin is in, or so the beauty culture tells us. By "beauty culture," we mean all those who are interested in telling us what our bodies should look like. This includes the diet, cosmetic, and fashion industries, and the media outlets that help disseminate the information provided by these industries. Many companies have a great interest in keeping us dissatisfied with our bodies. Companies don't spend advertising dollars to tell you that you're looking fine. No, they want you to see the need for their products. To sell a weight-loss diet, for instance, it is necessary to persuade customers that they are overweight. Skin and hair-care products find a market if they solve a perceived problem or fill a perceived need, such as the need for wrinkle-free skin no matter what your age. In addition, cosmetics and fashion industries ensure their futures by changing the styles each season. The beautiful fashions of today may well look ridiculous tomorrow; in time, they may then come back looking new and modern to another generation. Worse, the full lips that are so stylish one year (and can be attained through plastic surgery) may be replaced by thin lips the next. These changing standards of beauty, with their inevitable cycling, can only occur if the standards are arbitrary.

These industries aren't just selling diets and products, however; they're also selling ideas—ideas about how beauty is defined. When an idea and its attendant beauty products catch on, another idea is immediately put forward, with even more products to sell the new and improved beauty ideal. Even beyond the beauty-related industries, attractive bodies are used to sell all kinds of products. And, a better body is portrayed as the key to having fun, sex, intimacy, friends, family, and wealth. Why are these messages so effective? Well, if we heard only one of these messages it might seem ridiculous, but when we hear them over and over, we tend to believe them. The billion-dollar-per-year diet and beauty industry depends on our insecurity for its profits. About 8 percent of women are naturally a size ten, and our diet practically guarantees a population of even larger-sized people. The media presents smaller and smaller bodies, while the bodies of most of the population get larger.

A Balanced Response to the Beauty Culture

The media plays an important role in shaping our evaluation of our bodies. Some of us are more sensitive to these beauty culture messages, just as some are more sensitive to what our family members and friends think of us. The beauty culture provides a reference point with which we can compare ourselves. The ideal body seems so attainable, if only we used the right diet, cosmetic, or supplement.

Recognizing that our ideal body image is partly the result of clever marketing campaigns can encourage us to rebel and form our own ideas about what is beautiful or attractive. Do we really need to have someone else dictate our ideal body shape or size? It's time to accept and embrace the many wonderful variations of bodies, rather than strive to conform to the unrealistic ideals determined by the cosmetic, fashion, and diet industries. We are more valuable than our outer packaging. Our value lies in our minds and hearts, our skills and talents. Consider finding fulfillment in other areas. What can you do to fulfill dreams and meet goals not associated with body image? Changing your response to the beauty culture is the most powerful way you can take charge of your own body image.

We give power to our appearance that it doesn't deserve, power to determine our self-worth and what we do with our time and money. When we give appearance this much power, we blame it for every negative emotion and every unfortunate thing that happens to us. It grows in importance, becoming more significant than our abilities and talents in determining our self-worth. When our self-esteem dips, we may think we can fix the problem by starting a diet or buying a new outfit, cosmetic, or hair-care product. When this happens, delay making the purchase. Ask yourself why you are considering the expenditure: is this a beauty fix to help boost your self-esteem? We'll talk more about self-esteem in chapter 12.

Sometimes we come to believe that beauty can solve just about any problem. We may feel that life would be so much better if we were more attractive. We may even put off plans until we lose weight or otherwise improve our looks. Often we attribute the success of others and our own potential success to attractiveness. But how important is beauty? Good looks do tend to make a good first impression, but beyond that first impression there can be negatives. Attractive people often have to work hard to get beyond the stereotypes. "The dumb blonde" is a classic example. The actress who is deemed too thin and so is rumored to have an eating disorder is another example. So being beautiful or having the right kind of body doesn't solve every problem.

Changing our looks doesn't seem to actually help us *feel* more attractive. However, improving self-acceptance and self-esteem does. This helps us *feel* more attractive, and it makes us more confident and comfortable with ourselves and others. And that's attractive.

Cultural beauty messages set the stage for body-image dissatisfaction, but it is the importance we give these messages that contributes to the anxiety, stress, and depression associated with body-image problems. Beauty standards that are almost impossible to reach make it especially difficult to balance our own ideal body image with our perceived body image.

Mindless Response or Mindful Response?

Ellen Langer, Ph.D. (1990), has been studying the concept of mindfulness since the 1970s. She began with the study of *mindlessness*. She describes three forms of mindlessness. The first occurs when we rely too heavily on categories and distinctions that we've created in the past. Masculine or feminine, beautiful or ugly—categories that are too rigid can keep us seeing the world as black or white. Automatic behavior is the second form of mindlessness. We perform some activities while taking in and using only limited signals from the outside world, while ignoring other signals, saying excuse me when you bump into a store mannequin, for example. Habits can be the result of this type of mindlessness. The third form of mindlessness is acting from a single perspective, as if there were only one set of rules. This mindless attitude is at work when we assume strict standards of beauty or don't question our daily hair care, skin care, or diet.

In a sense, mindfulness is the opposite of mindlessness. Being mindful means continuously creating new categories: categorizing and re-categorizing, and labeling and relabeling. Instead of remembering a horrible childhood, for example, one might remember a childhood with both happy and sad experiences. When we are mindful, we are attentive to new information—especially important when we process the messages the beauty culture sends. When viewing advertisements, ask yourself some revealing questions: What are they really selling? Will it really do what it says? Is it worth it? What could I do with my money and time instead? What will I have to give up in order to purchase that product? Overtly, they are selling a product, but covertly, they are promising fun, happiness, friends, beauty, and sex. When you are mindful you know that the product cannot really deliver all this.

Being mindful means being open to different perspectives. Perhaps there is a different way to get ready for work in the morning, one that would take one hour instead of two. Perhaps Mary didn't ignore you but simply didn't see you, or perhaps John was upset about a problem at work, not bored by your company. Looking at different perspectives makes us more open to change. We can choose how to respond and act, rather than acting automatically. Question your motives. Is body image really that important to you, or are you just conditioned to give it importance?

But must we *always* be mindful of *everything*? Of course not; if we were our minds would be filled with jumbled thoughts—take a step, turn your head, open the door, and so on. The key is to know when to be mindful and when to be a bit mindless. There are times when studying a situation can increase our anxiety and waste our time on meaningless issues. And there are other times when examining a situation can shed lightly on it and inform us about how to respond. In the next few days, observe advertisements in a mindful way. Make several copies of the following worksheet to record your observations, or record them on a separate piece of paper. We've provided two completed worksheets as examples.

Healthy Respect and Care for the Body

Most experts agree that obesity makes a person more susceptible to a number of diseases, including heart disease, hypertension, and diabetes. Yo-yo dieting, losing and gaining weight over and over, also has negative effects on health and can lead to overall weight gain. Being slightly overweight, however, may actually have positive effects on health, such as reducing the incidence of heart disease and osteoporosis. Genetic makeup plays an important role in determining body size and shape. Compulsive exercise can exacerbate body dissatisfaction, but there is growing evidence that moderate exercise can lead to improvement of self-esteem, mood, and body satisfaction, in addition to providing health and fitness benefits. Exercise puts more focus on the performance, rather than appearance of the body.

With all this confusing and conflicting information, what should we do? Many people are inclined to do nothing, but this isn't the answer. A practical and realistic approach is to concentrate on taking care of your body. A healthy diet and moderate exercise will help you keep your body healthy, and a healthy body is an attractive body. Talk to your doctor and get his or her advice about choosing the healthy diet and exercise plan that is right for your body. Educate yourself about fitness—not thinness, but *fitness*. Understand that a person's weight is dependent on many factors, including genetics, psychological and social issues, and age. Enjoy manicures and pedicures, and indulge in the best hair-care products if you like, but also pay attention to other self-care measures: healthy eating, adequate sleep, relaxation, recreation, and spiritually uplifting activities. What self-care measures are you neglecting? List three ways you can take care of yourself this week—ways that don't have to do with appearance.

1. _____

2. _____

3. _____

Linda:

1. Eat more balanced meals; increase intake of fruits and vegetables.

2. Walk twenty minutes per day.

3. Go to a movie with a friend.

To some, changing their own response to the beauty culture might not seem like enough. It's true that we can't change the whole world, but we might be able to make some difference. Encourage others to look critically at advertisements. If you are offended by these ads or would like to see more varied body sizes and shapes, write and tell manufacturers. If a product doesn't fulfill its promises, write and complain. Refuse to buy from stores and catalogs that advertise in ways that perpetuate the myth of the perfect body. In your daily life, wear what you feel comfortable in. Talk to your friends and family members about your clothing and cosmetic choices, encourage and support others who choose to challenge current fashions, and stand up for those who are criticized. Together, we can make some changes. Even alone, we can feel that we've fought back against those who encourage us to remain dissatisfied with our bodies.

In the past, body-image dissatisfaction was thought of as a women's problem. Guys just weren't supposed to have eating disorders and body-image problems; naturally, men with these problems were reluctant to reveal their preoccupation with body image. In recent years our culture has helped increase the prevalence of body-image dissatisfaction, in both women and men. Fortunately, information about the problem is also more prevalent than it used to be. We'll discuss the effects of today's beauty culture on men in the next chapter.

Mindful Advertisement Observation

Advertisement #1

Describe the ad. _____

_____

What product is the advertiser selling? _____

What else do they seem to be selling? _____

_____

Even if the product fulfills its promise, is it worth the cost in time and money? What else could I do with that time and money if I didn't purchase this product? ____

_____

What subtle messages are hidden in the ad? _____

_____

Advertisement #2

Describe the ad. _____

_____

What product is the advertiser selling? _____

What else do they seem to be selling? _____

_____

Even if the product fulfills its promise, is it worth the cost in time and money? What else could I do with that time and money if I didn't purchase this product?

_____

What subtle messages are hidden in the ad? _____

_____

Mindful Advertisement Observation

Advertisement #1

Describe the ad. *A woman with clear, smooth skin. Her arms are folded and she looks happy, proud, and successful.*

What product is the advertiser selling? *Acne medicine.*

What else do they seem to be selling? *Success and pride. Not just getting rid of acne, but also smooth, clear skin.*

Even if the product fulfills its promise, is it worth the cost in time and money? What else could I do with that time and money if I didn't purchase this product? *It's probably not worth the money. Instead, I could buy several books, or pay a month's membership at a gym.*

What subtle messages are hidden in the ad? *You will look as beautiful as this girl and be happy and successful if you buy this product. People with clear skin are happy and beautiful.*

Advertisement #2

Describe the ad. *"Before" picture of a pale, frowning woman. "After" picture of the same woman, smiling, tan, blonder, fuller hair, thinner, and sucking in her stomach.*

What product is the advertiser selling? *Weight loss pills.*

What else do they seem to be selling? *Happier, brighter appearance when thinner.*

Even if the product fulfills its promise, is it worth the cost in time and money? What else could I do with that time and money if I didn't purchase this product? *Probably not worth the money. I could buy enough healthy food for 2 or 3 days for the price of one month's supply of diet pills.*

What subtle messages are hidden in the ad? *You could be thin like this woman, then you would be happy, smiling, and look more beautiful. Weight loss could make you look tanner and blonder.*

Mindful Advertisement Observation

Advertisement #1

Describe the ad. *Pretty, smiling girl with an arm around a handsome boy, pulling up the front of his shirt. The guy is laughing, very happy. American flag background.*

What product is the advertiser selling? *Cologne.*

What else do they seem to be selling? *Fun, happiness, beauty, intimacy, sexual attraction, patriotism.*

Even if the product fulfills its promise, is it worth the cost in time and money? What else could I do with that time and money if I didn't purchase this product? *This is an expensive cologne. A less expensive cologne would probably provide the same results. With that money I could probably buy a tank of gas or two shirts.*

What subtle messages are hidden in the ad? *If a guy uses this cologne, he can get the girl, have fun, and be patriotic. Attractive, fun people smell good.*

Advertisement #2

Describe the ad. *Sexy, smiling girl sitting on top of a giant pack of cigarettes in a desert setting.*

What product is the advertiser selling? *Cigarettes.*

What else do they seem to be selling? *Sexual attraction; maybe the possibility of getting a girl like that or looking like that girl.*

Even if the product fulfills its promise, is it worth the cost in time and money? What else could I do with that time and money if I didn't purchase this product? *Smoking would harm my health, so it's not worth it. I could buy a soda or a cup of coffee and still have money left over.*

What subtle messages are hidden in the ad? *Smoking is sexy and sophisticated.*

Chart 2c

CHAPTER 3

Muscle Dysmorphia and Other Male Body-Image Preoccupations

More and more men are becoming dissatisfied with their bodies. In a survey published in *Psychology Today* magazine in 1997, 43 percent of men reported dissatisfaction with their overall appearance. This demonstrated a dramatic increase, from 15 percent in 1972 and 34 percent in 1985. For women, overall appearance dissatisfaction had grown from 25 percent to 38 percent to 56 percent. Male body-image dissatisfaction is catching up with that of women.

Male Body Image, Yesterday and Today

Our world is changing. The same beauty culture that has depended on women's body dissatisfaction has recently targeted a new audience. Men are now bombarded with messages from the diet, fashion, fitness, and cosmetic industries. But don't blame only the advertisers and the beauty industries. It's really a two-way street—consumers' desire to look good, grow hair, gain muscle, and lose weight fuels these industries' growth. They are filling a need that our culture has created.

In the nineteenth century it was considered stylish for a man to be plump, if not fat. Plumpness was seen as an indication of wealth. Thinness represented poverty and poor nutrition. In the 1920s, the reverse became true: poor immigrants from southern and eastern Europe tended to be stocky and overweight, and so thinness and fitness were seen to represent wealth. In addition, movies were introduced at about that time. Thin bodies seemed to look best on film, and fitness was needed for action movies and Westerns. Like women, men saw the ideal body image on the movie screen (Luciano 2001).

Physical fitness began to receive more widespread attention in the 1950s. The President's Council on Youth Fitness, established in 1955, brought attention to the need for moderate exercise. Products appeared in the marketplace to help people exercise without effort. Some men and boys were attracted to bodybuilding, made popular by mail-order courses like the most famous one marketed by Charles Atlas. Fitness gained in popularity, and by the end of the 1960s Americans were spending millions of dollars every year on exercise equipment, such as treadmills and stationary bicycles. The 1970s saw the rise of aerobics, jogging, and health clubs, and clothing became more revealing than ever before. Bodybuilding gained popularity in the 1980s and continues to grow, as men strive to attain the muscular bodies they see in magazines and movies (Luciano 2001).

Even our children's playthings reflect the trend toward thinner and more muscular bodies. Barbie dolls have always celebrated the thin female body. She has gotten progressively thinner over the years; today, if she were a real woman, she would have a 16-inch waist. While Barbie has gotten thinner, G.I. Joe has become more muscular. The authors of *The Adonis Complex: The Secret Crisis of Male Body Obsession* (Pope, Phillips, and Olivardia 2000) compared the first G.I. Joes with today's. If he were a real man, the "G.I. Joe Land Adventurer" figure of 1964 would be five feet ten inches tall with a 32-inch waist, a 44-inch chest, and 12-inch biceps. The "Salute to G.I. Joe" figure of 1991 would have a 24-inch waist and 16½-inch biceps. G.I. Joe isn't alone; other play figures have also grown more muscular over the years.

Twenty percent of men have begun to lose their hair by their twenties and most have some male pattern baldness by age sixty. Hair loss is a normal process, yet men have fought it for centuries. Julius Caesar wore a ceremonial wreath to hide his receding hairline. From the fifteenth century into the eighteenth century, men wore wigs, which served as symbols of wealth and status. How ironic it is that men in the seventeenth century endeavored to appear older and wiser by wearing white powdered wigs, while men today want to appear younger than their actual age. Men wore wigs as status symbols in the past, but today they hide their wigs (Luciano 2001).

For centuries, men have also used various concoctions to stimulate hair growth. Egyptians used potions made of ibex, crocodile, and lion fat; human nail clippings; and singed hedgehog bristles as far back as 1,500 B.C. Hippocrates used opium mixed with floral essences, wine, and pigeon dung; Romans applied boiled snakes and painted hair on their balding heads. In seventeenth-century England, the rich applied a mixture of Indian tea and lemon to their heads, and the poor applied chicken droppings. The search for hair loss remedies continued into modern times. While nineteenth-century American settlers bought potions at fairs and medicine shows, Native Americans used yucca and chili-pepper oil. The pursuit of a cure for hair loss continues today (Luciano 2001).

Muscle Dysmorphia

Some people have nicknamed muscle dysmorphia "reverse anorexia" or "bigorexia nervosa." A subtype of body dysmorphic disorder, muscle dysmorphia is an excessive preoccupation with body size and muscularity. Instead of feeling fat when they're actually thin, people with this disorder feel small when they're actually big. They have obsessive thoughts that their muscles aren't big enough and feel puny and weak, even though they may actually have large, strong muscles.

In an attempt to reduce the obsessive thoughts and the related anxiety, people with muscle dysmorphia engage in compulsive behaviors to try to increase muscle mass. Even when weightlifting, taking diet supplements, and sometimes ingesting dangerous substances increase their muscle size, they often don't see the growth. Instead, they continue to see a thin, puny, weak person staring back from the mirror. This perception leads to an ongoing cycle of obsessive thoughts and compulsive behaviors. What causes this cycle? Most likely, three factors are responsible. First is a probable genetic predisposition to obsessive-compulsive behavior. Second is the way we react emotionally to our upbringing, childhood teasing, and other personal experiences. Third is the important part our culture plays in fueling the feelings of inadequacy.

There seem to be more cases of muscle dysmorphia today than in the past. Why? People with a predisposition to obsessive-compulsive symptoms may have focused more on things like checking door locks or hand washing in the past; our image-oriented culture has probably led to an increase in the number of people who focus their obsessive-compulsive behavior on appearance. Are we saying all bodybuilding is harmful? Of course not—it's healthy to exercise. Only when it is a preoccupation, or is associated with distress, anxiety, or impaired functioning, does it become unhealthy and harmful. We can compare it to hand washing. Not washing your hands at all is unhealthy, but so is washing your hands one hundred times a day. Working out is healthy, but when done in excess it can be a disorder. Ask yourself the following questions.

1. Are you preoccupied with thoughts that your body is not lean or muscular enough?

2. Does weightlifting or diet management interfere with your family life, job, or recreational activities?

3. Do you avoid situations where your body would be exposed to others, or are you very anxious when you must be exposed?

4. Do you continue to work out, diet, or use supplements even when there is evidence these behaviors are causing physical or psychological harm?

5. Are you using anabolic steroids? (If your answer to this question is "yes," you need to seek medical attention.)

If you answered "yes" to any of these questions, you need to consider that you may have a body-image problem and possibly muscle dysmorphia. You could probably benefit from both professional help and the Balanced Image Program.

The Danger of Anabolic Steroids

German scientists discovered testosterone, the primary male hormone, in the 1930s. They developed *analogs* of testosterone, drugs with slight chemical changes to the testosterone molecule. These drugs are called *anabolic-androgenic steroids*. Experimentation with these drugs led to the discovery in the 1950s that they could increase muscle mass and strength. Bodybuilders and athletes had found the secret to growing big, muscled shoulders and arms.

At first, it remained a secret in the sports world. Athletes with progressively larger muscles began to appear on the scene, and male sports fans were led to believe that the muscles were the result of improved dietary supplements and training techniques, dedication, and persistence. Many men struggled to attain bodies they could never achieve alone. In the 1980s, many male actors and models began to show signs of "'roided" bodies. The secret was gradually revealed, and more men and boys became tempted to use steroids in order to attain the kinds of bodies they saw in magazines and movies. Anabolic steroids may be used legally to treat conditions in which the body produces abnormally low amounts of testosterone, such as delayed puberty and some types of impotence, or to treat body wasting in patients with AIDS. They are used illegally by bodybuilders, athletes, and others enticed by the promise of enhanced athletic performance or increased muscle size.

Steroid use puts one at greater risk of developing heart disease, stroke, and possibly prostate cancer. The biggest dangers are the psychiatric side effects, however extreme mood swings, insomnia, irritability, and aggression can occur. These can progress to paranoid jealousy, extreme irritability, delusions, impaired judgement, and feelings of invincibility. Severe depression can develop during withdrawal, and this can lead to further drug use. Some users go on to use other illegal drugs in an effort to lessen the side effects of the steroids.

A term has been coined to describe violence, hostility, and antisocial behavior that can result from steroid use: "'roid rage." Not everyone who uses steroids will experience 'roid rage. Because these severe reactions aren't always reported, we don't know how often they occur. While a person is more likely to experience 'roid rage when taking steroids at high doses, rages have been reported to occur in people taking low doses. At least twenty cases of murder and numerous cases of domestic violence, child abuse, assaults, and suicide have been linked to the use of anabolic steroids in the United States. Ironically, studies have shown that a greater percentage of women prefer men with normal-looking muscles over big, muscled hunks. For a thorough discussion of muscle dysmorphia and male body obsession, read *The Adonis Complex: The Secret Crisis of Male Body Obsession* by Harrison G. Pope Jr., M.D., Katharine A. Phillips, M.D., and Roberto Olivardia, Ph.D.

Now that you've learned about male body-image dissatisfaction, review chapter 1, especially the discussion about the balanced response to the beauty culture. Complete several Mindful Advertisement Observation worksheets. The next chapter will help you better understand body-image dissatisfaction and will introduce you to body dysmorphic disorder.

CHAPTER 4

Do I Have BDD?

How do you know if you have body dysmorphic disorder or a related problem, or simply a little concern over your body image? In this chapter we will ask you to complete a couple of questionnaires and respond to some questions about yourself. We'll help you figure out what the answers mean. Lilly's responded to the same questions are included as examples. The questions are derived from measures used by researchers looking at BDD and related problems. The first is the Body Dysmorphic Disorder Questionnaire, which was devised by Katharine Phillips, M.D., researcher, author of *The Broken Mirror: Understanding and Treating Body Dysmorphic Disorder*, and coauthor of *The Adonis Complex: The Secret Crisis of Male Body Obsessions*

The Body Dysmorphic Disorder Questionnaire (BDDQ)*

This questionnaire assesses concerns about physical appearance. Please read each question carefully and circle the answer that best describes your experience. Also write in answers where indicated.

1. Are you worried about how you look?   Yes   No

   —If yes: Do you think about your appearance problems a lot
   and wish you could think about them less?   Yes   No

   —If yes: Please list the body areas you don't like. _____

   _____

   _____

   Examples of disliked body areas include: your skin (for example, acne, scars, wrinkles, paleness, redness); hair; the shape or size of your nose, mouth, jaw, lips, stomach, hips, etc.; or defects of your hands, genitals, breasts, or any other body part.

NOTE: If you answered "No" to either of the above questions, you are finished with this questionnaire. Otherwise continue.

2. Is your *main* concern with how you look that you aren't thin enough
   or that you might get too fat?   Yes   No

3. How has this problem with how you look affected your life?

   • Has it often upset you a lot?   Yes   No

   • Has it often gotten in the way of doing things with friends
     or dating?   Yes   No

     —If yes: Describe how. _____

     _____

* The Body Dysmorphic Disorder Questionnaire (BDDQ), from *The Broken Mirror: Understanding and Treating Body Dysmorphic Disorder*, by Katharine A. Phillips, M.D., 1996 (revised). Used with permission from the author.

- Has it caused you any problems with school or work?   Yes   No

  —If yes: What are they? _____

  _____

- Are there things you avoid because of how you look?   Yes   No

  —If yes: What are they? _____

  _____

4. On an average day, how much time do you usually spend thinking about how you look? (Add up all the time you spend, then circle one.)

(a) Less than 1 hour a day   (b) 1–3 hours a day   (c) More than 3 hours a day

Lilly's Answers to The Body Dysmorphic Disorder Questionnaire (BDDQ)

This questionnaire assesses concerns about physical appearance. Please read each question carefully and circle the answer that best describes your experience. Also write in answers where indicated.

1. Are you worried about how you look?   (Yes) No

   —If yes: Do you think about your appearance problems a lot and wish you could think about them less?   (Yes) No

   —If yes: Please list the body areas you don't like. _____
   My thighs and my stomach. _____

   Examples of disliked body areas include: your skin (for example, acne, scars, wrinkles, paleness, redness); hair; the shape or size of your nose, mouth, jaw, lips, stomach, hips, etc.; or defects of your hands, genitals, breasts, or any other body part.

NOTE: If you answered "No" to either of the above questions, you are finished with this questionnaire. Otherwise continue.

2. Is your *main* concern with how you look that you aren't thin enough or that you might get too fat?   Yes (No)

3. How has this problem with how you look affected your life?

   - Has it often upset you a lot?   (Yes) No

   - Has it often gotten in the way of doing things with friends or dating?   (Yes) No

   —If yes: Describe how. *When I do go out, I change clothes over and over, and then I decide to wear something loose fitting that won't show my fat thighs and stomach so much. I hate to go any place where I might see l people I know. I avoid sex and am embarrassed to let my husband see me without clothes. I know he is worried about me. Old friends wonder why I won't see them.*

- Has it caused you any problems with school or work?   Yes No

—If yes: What are they? *I spend a lot of time in the bathroom checking myself in the mirror and changing clothes. I don't pay as much attention to my kids as I'd like because I'm always thinking about my thighs and stomach.*

- Are there things you avoid because of how you look?   Yes No

—If yes: What are they? *I avoid people who might judge my appearance negatively, clothes that would show my figure, and mirrors, to keep from getting upset. Other times, I check myself in mirrors over and over.*

4. On an average day, how much time do you usually spend thinking about how you look? (Add up all the time you spend, then circle one.)

(a) Less than 1 hour a day   (b) 1–3 hours a day (c) More than 3 hours a day

Let's take a look at your answers and Lilly's answers. We told you to stop if your answers to both parts of question 1 were "no." This question asks if you are *preoccupied* with a defect. If you aren't preoccupied, you don't have BDD. Terms like *preoccupied* may be hard to define precisely, but most people who do have BDD would agree that they are preoccupied. Question 2 helps separate out people who may have an eating disorder instead. As we explained in chapter 1, eating disorders are considered to be different from BDD, although these two types of disorders are probably related and have many overlapping features. It is possible for people to have both an eating disorder and BDD, but the defect that is the focus of concern would be something other than weight. Although this book is written for people who have BDD and similar body-image concerns, people with eating disorders such as anorexia nervosa may also find it helpful to answer the questions and do the exercises in this book.

Lilly did diet and exercise to try to lose weight, but not because of her overall appearance; she did so only to reduce the size of her thighs and stomach, which she thought were much too large. She readily admitted that her weight was well within normal limits, but she considered weight loss a kind of necessary side effect of making her thighs and stomach look right.

Question 3 addresses the effects of your preoccupation on your life. The *DSM-IV-TR* diagnostic criteria for BDD, which are meant to be guidelines and are not chiseled in stone, call for the preoccupation to cause *clinically significant* distress or impairment of social, occupational, or other important functioning (APA 2000). Like the word *preoccupied*, the phrase *clinically significant* is hard to define precisely. If you answered "yes" to any part of question 3, then your body-image problem is significant enough for you to consider self-help treatment through the Balanced Image Program (see chapters 7 through 15). Review your answers to question 3: you are in the best position to decide whether your distress or impairment meets the standard of clinically significant.

Lilly had no doubts that her preoccupation with the appearance of her thighs and stomach greatly impaired her ability to function in every part of her life. She was thinking about her appearance almost every waking minute. She would spend hours checking herself in the mirror and changing clothes, and just as many hours poring over magazines to find ways to change her appearance and comparing her stomach and thighs with those of the models.

Question 4 helps you look at the severity of your body-image problem. Most people with BDD would probably answer that they spend more than an hour a day preoccupied with or thinking about their defect(s). At first, Lilly didn't think she spent three hours a day thinking about the appearance of her thighs and stomach. But after a day of listening to her own thoughts, she realized she was spending well over three hours a day, maybe closer to six or eight. The thoughts seemed to be always with her.

People who do not have BDD, but who do have dissatisfaction with their body image, generally spend much less time being preoccupied, and the effects on their lives are less severe. If you still aren't sure whether your body-image concerns are severe enough for you to need help, consider a couple more questions: Why did you pick up this book? Would your life be more productive or fulfilling if you spent less time concerned about your body image? If your answer to the second question is "yes," you may have a significant problem with body image.

We will take a closer look at the amount of time you spend focusing on your defect in the next questionnaire, which will help you assess the severity of your problem. You may notice that none of the questions asks whether the defect is imagined, whether the reactions are markedly excessive. This is because many people with body-image dissatisfaction would answer questions like these by simply denying that their defect is imagined and saying that their reactions are not out of proportion.

Most people with body-image dissatisfaction have already asked others about their appearance and have been told that they look fine or that the problem is really minimal. If you've already sought this reassurance you know it only seems to help for a little while, if at all. You may think that others are just trying to be nice or make you feel better. Whatever defects in appearance you may have, the best choice is to accept that you don't look the way you want to and work on reducing the importance of your appearance. Instead of trying to find ways to fix or hide the defect or seek convincing evidence that your appearance is satisfactory, you can explore ways to cope with defects and learn to live life fully and happily, regardless of what you look like. Of course, we aren't saying that reasonable efforts to improve appearance are wrong. The key word here is *reasonable*. We want to help you move from being preoccupied to accepting.

Getting a Better Understanding of Your Body-Image Dissatisfaction

Next, let's look at another set of questions to help you understand your appearance concerns. Dr. James Rosen, a leading researcher on BDD and related disorders at the University of Vermont, developed the following questionnaire. It was designed to measure the severity of body dysmorphic disorder symptoms.

Body Dysmorphic Disorder Examination—
Self Report (BDDE-SR)*

Part 1

1. In the *first* column below, please check up to *five parts* of your physical appearance that you've disliked the most (or at least have not been completely satisfied with) during the past month. *Be as specific as possible,* choosing the term that *best describes* the body area you have in mind.

2. In the *second* column, describe what is dissatisfying about it. For example, if "nose" was checked in the first column, you might write "It's too big" in the second. If there is more than one reason you are dissatisfied with the part, please list each reason (e.g., thighs might be "too big" and also "have fat dimples").

3. In the *third* column, please *rank order* how dissatisfying the body part(s) checked are. Assign a "1" to the most dissatisfying body part, a "2" to the second most dissatisfying, etc. Please do not rank more than 5 body parts.

Check 5 part(s) you are dissatisfied with	What don't you like about it?	Rank most to least dissatisfying; 1=most
feet _____	_____	_____
calves _____	_____	_____
thighs _____	_____	_____
entire leg(s) _____	_____	_____
butt _____	_____	_____
hips _____	_____	_____
all lower body _____	_____	_____
waist abdomen _____	_____	_____
chest _____	_____	_____
breasts _____	_____	_____
back _____	_____	_____
shoulders _____	_____	_____
all upper body _____	_____	_____
back of arm _____	_____	_____
entire arm(s) _____	_____	_____
hands _____	_____	_____
whole body _____	_____	_____
neck _____	_____	_____
genitals _____	_____	_____
chin _____	_____	_____
cheeks _____	_____	_____

* Body Dysmorphic Disorder Examination—Self Report (BDDE-SR) by James C. Rosen, Ph.D., and Jeff Reiter, Ph.D. Version #3, 1994. Used with permission from authors.

mouth   _____   _____   _____

teeth   _____   _____   _____

nose   _____   _____   _____

eyes   _____   _____   _____

eyebrows   _____   _____   _____

ears   _____   _____   _____

facial hair   _____   _____   _____

whole face   _____   _____   _____

body hair   _____   _____   _____

head hair   _____   _____   _____

OTHER   _____   please describe   _____

                         _____

OTHER   _____   please describe   _____

                         _____

Part 2

Listed below are things people sometimes try in order to change or improve their appearance. Please indicate any that you have tried for the sake of improving the appearance of the *BODY PART YOU RATED AS "1"* (that is, the most dissatisfying part) on the previous list. *INCLUDE EVERYTHING YOU'VE TRIED,* not just what you've tried in the past four weeks. Please estimate how many times you have tried the method. *DO NOT* include a remedy that you may have used for an appearance concern unrelated to the one you rated as "1" (for example, do not include cosmetic surgery for your nose if you did not rate your nose as "1" above).

Number of Times Tried	**Remedy**
_____	A specific diet to improve appearance
_____	A specific exercise program to improve appearance
_____	Surgery to reduce weight (e.g., stomach stapling or bypass)
_____	Cosmetic surgery (e.g., liposuction, breast reduction or implants, nose job, scar revision, facelift, collagen for lips)
_____	Nonsurgical dental work (e.g., braces, teeth whitening)
_____	Ointments or medications (for skin conditions or baldness)
_____	Hair transplant
_____	Prosthesis (e.g., artificial leg; only include this if one reason for getting it was to improve appearance)
_____	Other (please describe in the space below, including number of times tried)

_____

_____

Part 3

1. Before working on these questions, be sure you completed Parts 1 and 2 of the BDDE-SR answer form.

2. The following questions will ask you to think about your "appearance feature"— this refers to the body part you ranked as number "1" on the list. Answer according to the past four weeks.

3. To answer the questions, you may choose any number from 0 to 6, even if there is no description next to it. Record your answers on the answer form (see page 55).

Over the past four weeks:

1. How common have you felt it is for people your age and sex to have an appearance feature just like the one you believe you have?

   0—everyone has the same feature
   1—
   2—many people have the same feature
   3—
   4—few people have the same feature
   5—
   6—no one else has the same feature (or the extent of the problem in others is not as severe)

2. How frequently have you checked out your appearance feature (for example, looked at it, felt it, measured it in some way) in order to evaluate the extent of the problem?

   0—(0 days) no checking
   1—(1–3 days)
   2—(4–7 days) checking once or twice a week
   3—(8–11 days)
   4—(12–16 days) checking on about half the days
   5—(17–21 days)
   6—(22–28 days) checking every or almost every day

3. How dissatisfied have you been with your appearance feature?

   0—no dissatisfaction
   1—
   2—slight dissatisfaction (but no feelings of distress)
   3—
   4—moderate dissatisfaction (with some feelings of distress)
   5—
   6—extreme dissatisfaction (with extreme distress; could not imagine feeling more upset or dissatisfied)

4. How dissatisfied have you been with your overall appearance?

   0—no dissatisfaction
   1—
   2—slight dissatisfaction (but no feelings of distress)
   3—

4—moderate dissatisfaction (with some feelings of distress)

5—

6—extreme dissatisfaction (with extreme distress; can't imagine feeling more dissatisfied)

5. How frequently have you tried to get reassurance from someone that your appearance feature isn't as bad or abnormal as you think it is?

0—(0 days) never sought reassurance

1—(1–3 days)

2—(4–7 days) sought reassurance once or twice a week

3—(8–11 days)

4—(12–16 days) sought reassurance on about half the days

5—(17–21 days)

6—(22–28 days) sought reassurance every or almost every day

6. How often have you thought about your appearance feature AND felt upset as a result?

0—(0 days) never think about the appearance feature with upset feelings

1—(1–3 days)

2—(4–7 days) think about it and feel upset once or twice a week

3—(8–11 days)

4—(12–16 days) think about it and feel upset on about half the days

5—(17–21 days)

6—(22–28 days) think about it and feel upset every or almost every day

7. How much have you worried or felt embarrassed about your appearance feature when you were in public areas such as shopping malls, grocery stores, city streets, restaurants, movies, clubs, buses or planes, waiting in lines, parks or beaches, public restrooms, or other areas where mainly there were people you didn't know? (When answering, think about how many of these situations you worry in and how intense your worrying is.)

0—no worrying or embarrassment

1—

2—slight amount of worrying or embarrassment

3—

4—moderate amount of worrying or embarrassment

5—

6—extreme worrying or embarrassment

8. How much have you worried or felt embarrassed about your appearance feature when you were in social settings with co-workers, acquaintances, friends, or family members (for example, at work, parties, family gatherings, meetings, talking in groups, having a conversation, dating or going on an outing with others, speaking to a boss or supervisor)?

0—no worrying or embarrassment

1—

2—slight amount of worrying or embarrassment

3—

4—moderate amount of worrying or embarrassment

5—

6—extreme worrying or embarrassment

9a. How often have you felt that other people were noticing or paying attention to your appearance feature? (Include times when you realize you might be imagining it.)

0—(0 days) never occurred
1—(1–3 days)
2—(4–7 days) occurred once or twice a week
3—(8–11 days)
4—(12–16 days) occurred on about half the days
5—(17–21 days)
6—(22–28 days) occurred every or almost every day

9b. How upset have you become when you felt someone was noticing or paying attention to your appearance feature? (When answering, think about whether you feel differently depending on who the person is that notices.)

0—not upsetting (or others do not notice)
1—slightly upsetting when certain people are involved, but not others
2—slightly upsetting regardless of who is involved
3—moderately upsetting when certain people are involved, but not others
4—moderately upsetting regardless of who is involved
5—extremely upsetting when certain people are involved but not others
6—extremely upsetting regardless of who is involved

10a. How often has someone unexpectedly made a positive or negative comment on your appearance feature? (Only include comments that came "out of the blue," not comments you might have tried to get from the person.)

0—(0 days) never occurred
1—(1–3 days)
2—(4–7 days) occurred once or twice a week
3—(8–11 days)
4—(12–16 days) occurred on about half the days
5—(17–21 days)
6—(22–28 days) occurred every or almost every day

10b. How upset have you become when someone commented—positively or negatively—on your appearance feature? (When answering, think about whether you feel differently depending on who the person is that made the comment.)

0—not upsetting (or others did not comment)
1—slightly upsetting when certain people commented, but not others
2—slightly upsetting regardless of who commented
3—moderately upsetting when certain people commented, but not others
4—moderately upsetting regardless of who commented
5—extremely upsetting when certain people commented, but not others
6—extremely upsetting regardless of who commented

11a. How often has someone done something to you or for you that you think is a result of your appearance feature.

0—(0 days) never occurred
1—(1–3 days)

2—(4–7 days) occurred once or twice a week
3—(8–11 days)
4—(12–16 days) occurred on about half the days
5—(17–21 days)
6—(22–28 days) occurred every or almost every day

11b. How upset have you become when someone has done something to you or for you, because of your appearance feature? (When answering, think about whether you feel differently depending on who the person is.)

0—not upsetting (or others did not treat me differently)
1—slightly upsetting when certain people were involved, but not others
2—slightly upsetting regardless of who was involved
3—moderately upsetting when certain people were involved, but not others
4—moderately upsetting regardless of who was involved
5—extremely upsetting when certain people were involved, but not others
6—extremely upsetting regardless of who was involved

12. How important has appearance been in how you evaluate yourself as a person? Before answering, think about other things that influence how you judge yourself—such as personality, intelligence, work or school performance, quality of your relationships with others, ability in other areas, and so on. Compared to these (and maybe others), how much importance have you given to appearance when evaluating yourself?

0—no importance
1—
2—some importance (definitely an aspect of self-evaluation)
3—
4—moderate importance (one of the main aspects of self-evaluation)
5—
6—extreme importance (nothing is more important as a means of evaluating yourself)

13. How negatively have you thought of yourself as a person as a result of your appearance feature? This question is not asking whether you think your appearance is attractive or unattractive. Rather, it is asking how much your appearance made you feel that you had a personal flaw or were undesirable or inadequate in a *non-physical* way.

0—no negative evaluations of yourself resulting from your appearance feature
1—
2—slightly negative evaluations of yourself
3—
4—moderately negative evaluations of yourself
5—
6—extremely negative evaluations of yourself; the appearance feature makes you unable to find positive qualities in yourself

14. How negatively (if at all) have you felt *other* people evaluated you as a person as a result of your appearance feature? Again, this question is not asking how attractive or unattractive other people think you are. Rather it is asking how much you think your appearance made other people see you as undesirable or inadequate in some *non-physical* way.

0—no negative evaluations by others resulting from your appearance feature
1—
2—slightly negative evaluations by others
3—
4—moderately negative evaluations by others
5—
6—extremely negative evaluations by others; the appearance feature makes others unable to find positive qualities in you

15. How attractive physically do you feel other people thought you were? (If friends view you differently than strangers, how attractive *on average* do you feel people think you are?)

0—attractive, or at least not unattractive
1—
2—slightly unattractive
3—
4—moderately unattractive
5—
6—extremely unattractive

16a. Have you ever thought your appearance feature might not be as bad as you generally think or have there been times that you've felt significantly better about your appearance feature?

       yes _____   no _____

16b. Have you ever felt during the past month that your appearance is basically normal?

       yes _____   no _____

17. How much have you avoided *public areas* because you felt uncomfortable about your appearance feature? (Such areas might include shopping malls, grocery stores, city streets, restaurants, movies, clubs, buses or planes, waiting in lines, parks or beaches, public restrooms, or other areas where mainly there would be *people you don't know.*)

0—no avoidance of public situations
1—
2—avoided with slight frequency
3—
4—avoided with moderate frequency
5—
6—avoided with extreme frequency

18. How much have you avoided *work or other social situations* with friends, relatives, or acquaintances because you felt uncomfortable about your appearance feature? Social situations could include going to work or school, parties, family gatherings, meetings, talking in groups, having a conversation, hanging out with others at work, dating or going on an outing with others, speaking to a boss or supervisor.

0—no avoidance of social situations
1—
2—avoided with slight frequency
3—

4—avoided with moderate frequency
5—
6—avoided with extreme frequency

19. How much have you avoided close physical contact with others because of your appearance feature? This includes sexual activity as well as other close contact such as shaking hands, hugging, kissing, or dancing close.

0—no avoidance of physical contact
1—
2—avoided with slight frequency
3—
4—avoided with moderate frequency
5—
6—avoided with extreme frequency

20. When making contact physically with others (for example, lovemaking, hugging, shaking hands, kissing, dancing close), how often have you tried to restrict the amount of actual contact that occurs (for example, by changing your posture, limiting your movement, or preventing contact with certain body parts)?

0—never deliberately restricted physical contact
1—
2—restricted on less than half the physical contact occasions
3—
4—restricted on about half the physical contact occasions
5—
6—restricted on every or almost every physical contact occasion

21. How much have you avoided physical activities such as exercise or outdoor recreation because of feeling self-conscious or uncomfortable due to your appearance feature?

0—no avoidance of physical activity
1—
2—avoided with slight frequency
3—
4—avoided with moderate frequency
5—
6—avoided with extreme frequency

22. How much have you deliberately dressed, made yourself up, or groomed yourself in some special way in order to cover up your appearance feature or distract attention from it? (This can include *avoiding* certain clothes or cosmetics.) This is called "camouflaging."

0—(0 days) never camouflaged or avoided certain clothes/cosmetics
1—(1–3 days)
2—(4–7 days) camouflaged once or twice a week
3—(8–11 days)
4—(12–16 days) camouflaged on about half the days
5—(17–21 days)
6—(22–28 days) camouflaged every or almost every day

23. How frequently have you deliberately changed your posture or body movements (such as the way you stand or sit, where you put your hands, how you walk, what side of yourself you show to other people, etc.) in order to hide your appearance feature or distract people's attention from it?

    0—(0 days) no changing of posture or body movements
    1—(1–3 days)
    2—(4–7 days) changed once or twice a week
    3—(8–11 days)
    4—(12–16 days) changed on about half the days
    5—(17–21 days)
    6—(22–28 days) changed every or almost every day

24. How often have you avoided looking at your body, particularly at your appearance feature, in order to control feelings about your appearance? This includes avoiding looking at yourself clothed or unclothed either directly or in mirrors or windows.

    0—(0 days) never avoided looking at body
    1—(1–3 days)
    2—(4–7 days) avoided once or twice a week
    3—(8–11 days)
    4—(12–16 days) avoided on about half the days
    5—(17–21 days)
    6—(22–28 days) avoided every or almost every day

25. How frequently have you avoided other people seeing your body unclothed because you felt uncomfortable about your appearance feature? This includes not letting your spouse, partner, roommate, etc., see you without clothes, or people in public settings such as in health club showers or changing rooms.

    0—no avoidance of others seeing body unclothed
    1—
    2—avoided with slight frequency
    3—
    4—avoided with moderate frequency
    5—
    6—avoided with extreme frequency

26. How often have you compared your appearance with the appearance of other people around you or in magazines or television? Include both positive and negative comparisons.

    0—(0 days) no comparing with others
    1—(1–3 days)
    2—(4–7 days) compared once or twice a week
    3—(8–11 days)
    4—(12–16 days) compared on about half the days
    5—(17–21 days)
    6—(22–28 days) compared every or almost every day

Circle the best answer to the questions above.

1. 0	1	2	3	4	5	6	13. 0	1	2	3	4	5	6
2. 0	1	2	3	4	5	6	14. 0	1	2	3	4	5	6
3. 0	1	2	3	4	5	6	15. 0	1	2	3	4	5	6
4. 0	1	2	3	4	5	6	16a. yes	no					
5. 0	1	2	3	4	5	6	16b. yes	no					
6. 0	1	2	3	4	5	6	17. 0	1	2	3	4	5	6
7. 0	1	2	3	4	5	6	18. 0	1	2	3	4	5	6
8. 0	1	2	3	4	5	6	19. 0	1	2	3	4	5	6
9a. 0	1	2	3	4	5	6	20. 0	1	2	3	4	5	6
9b. 0	1	2	3	4	5	6	21. 0	1	2	3	4	5	6
10a. 0	1	2	3	4	5	6	22. 0	1	2	3	4	5	6
10b. 0	1	2	3	4	5	6	23. 0	1	2	3	4	5	6
11a. 0	1	2	3	4	5	6	24. 0	1	2	3	4	5	6
11b. 0	1	2	3	4	5	6	25. 0	1	2	3	4	5	6
12. 0	1	2	3	4	5	6	26. 0	1	2	3	4	5	6

Scoring Part 3

First add up your answers for questions 1 to 15 and write the sum here. _____

Next add up your answers for questions 17 to 26 and write the sum here. _____

Put your total score here. _____

1. Did you score yourself 4 or higher on items 6, 12, and 13?   Yes No

2. Did you score yourself 4 or higher on items 7 or 8?   Yes No

3. Did you score yourself 4 or higher on items 9b, 17, 18, 19 or 21?   Yes No

Lilly's Answers to Body Dysmorphic Disorder Examination—Self Report (BDDE-SR)

Part 1

1. In the *first* column below, please check up to *five parts* of your physical appearance that you've disliked the most (or at least have not been completely satisfied with) during the past month. *Be as specific as possible,* choosing the term that *best describes* the body area you have in mind.

2. In the *second* column describe what is dissatisfying about it. For example, if "nose" was checked in the first column, you might write "It's too big" in the second. If there is more than one reason you are dissatisfied with the part, please list each reason (e.g., thighs might be "too big" and also "have fat dimples").

3. In the *third* column, please *rank order* how dissatisfying the body part(s) checked are. Assign a "1" to the most dissatisfying body part, a "2" to the second most dissatisfying, etc. Please do not rank more than 5 body parts.

Check 5 part(s) you are dissatisfied with		What don't you like about it?	Rank most to least dissatisfying; 1=most
feet	_____	_____	_____
calves	_____	_____	_____
thighs	_X_	_too fat, misshapen,_	
		lumpy, grotesque	_1_
entire leg(s)	_____	_____	_____
butt	_X_	_lumpy, fat_	_4_
hips	_X_	_misshapen, lumpy,_	
		fat, ugly	_3_
all lower body	_____	_____	_____
waist abdomen	_X_	_stomach sticks out_	
		too much; fat	_2_
chest	_____	_____	_____
breasts	_____	_____	_____
back	_____	_____	_____
shoulders	_____	_____	_____
all upper body	_____	_____	_____
back of arm	_____	_____	_____
entire arm(s)	_____	_____	_____
hands	_____	_____	_____
whole body	_____	_____	_____
neck	_____	_____	_____
genitals	_____	_____	_____
chin	_____	_____	_____
cheeks	_____	_____	_____
mouth	_____	_____	_____
teeth	_____	_____	_____
nose	_____	_____	_____
eyes	_____	_____	_____
eyebrows	_____	_____	_____
ears	_____	_____	_____
facial hair	_____	_____	_____
whole face	_____	_____	_____
body hair	_____	_____	_____
head hair	_____	_____	_____
OTHER	_____	please describe	_____
		_____	
OTHER	_____	please describe	_____
		_____	

Part 2

Listed below are things people sometimes try in order to change or improve their appearance. Please indicate any that you have tried for the sake of improving the appearance of the *BODY PART YOU RATED AS "1"* (that is, the most dissatisfying part) on the previous list. *INCLUDE EVERYTHING YOU'VE TRIED,* not just what you've tried in the past four weeks. Please estimate how many times you have tried the method. *DO NOT* include a remedy that you may have used for an appearance concern unrelated to the one you rated as "1" (for example, do not include cosmetic surgery for your nose if you did not rate your nose as "1" above).

Number of Times Tried	Remedy
_15_	A specific diet to improve appearance
_20_	A specific exercise program to improve appearance
_____	Surgery to reduce weight (e.g., stomach stapling or bypass)
_____	Cosmetic surgery (e.g., liposuction, breast reduction or implants, nose job, scar revision, facelift, collagen for lips)
_____	Nonsurgical dental work (e.g., braces, teeth whitening)
_5_	Ointments or medications (for skin conditions or baldness)
_____	Hair transplant
_____	Prosthesis (e.g., artificial leg; only include this if one reason for getting it was to improve appearance)
_20_	Other (please describe in the space below, including number of times tried)

Clothing to hide my fat thighs and stomach. Styles to make them look smaller and less deformed looking.

Circle the best answer to the questions above.

1. 0	1	2	③	4	5	6	13. 0	1	2	3	4	⑤	6
2. 0	1	2	3	4	5	⑥	14. 0	1	2	3	④	5	6
3. 0	1	2	3	4	⑤	6	15. 0	1	2	3	④	5	6
4. 0	1	2	3	④	5	6	16a. ⟨yes⟩ no						
5. 0	1	2	3	④	5	6	16b. yes ⟨no⟩						
6. 0	1	2	3	4	⑤	6	17. 0	1	2	③	4	5	6
7. 0	1	2	3	④	5	6	18. 0	1	2	3	4	⑤	6
8. 0	1	2	3	4	⑤	6	19. 0	1	2	3	④	5	6
9a. 0	1	2	3	④	5	6	20. 0	1	2	3	4	⑤	6
9b. 0	1	2	3	④	5	6	21. 0	1	2	3	④	5	6
10a. 0	①	2	3	4	5	6	22. 0	1	2	3	4	5	⑥
10b. 0	1	2	3	④	5	6	23. 0	1	2	3	4	⑤	6
11a. 0	1	②	3	4	5	6	24. 0	1	2	3	④	5	6
11b. 0	1	2	3	④	5	6	25. 0	1	2	3	4	⑤	6
12. 0	1	2	3	4	⑤	6	26. 0	1	2	3	4	⑤	6

Scoring Part 3

First add up your answers for questions 1 to 15 and write the sum here.   _73_

Next add up your answers for questions 17 to 26 and write the sum here.   _46_

Put your total score here.   _119_

1. Did you score yourself 4 or higher on items 6, 12, and 13?   (Yes) No

2. Did you score yourself 4 or higher on items 7 or 8?   (Yes) No

3. Did you score yourself 4 or higher on items 9b, 17, 18, 19 or 21?   (Yes) No

One of the diagnostic criteria for BDD is that the preoccupation causes clinically significant distress or impairment in social, occupational, or other important areas of functioning. If you answered "yes" to questions 1 and 2, you indicated clinically significant distress. If you answered "yes" to question 3, you indicated interference with functioning. These are signs of a problem. If what you consider a defect is something others don't see at all, or if others see your concern as markedly excessive, and if you don't have another disorder or problem such as anorexia nervosa that would explain your concern, then you are likely to have BDD.

During preparation of the BDDE-SR, Dr. Rosen's research samples showed that among college students males scored an average of about 33 and females about 50 on the BDDE-SR. Among people seeking treatment for body-image problems, the average score for males was about 99 and for women 89. Since these are average scores, there were many people in each group who scored higher or lower. There is no magic number or specific score that indicates you do or don't have a problem. Try to think of your score as giving you a way to see where you are now. As you work on the Balanced Image Program in this book you can answer the same questions again and see how you have changed.

Below is one more questionnaire that has been widely used in research and is considered the standard measure of the severity of BDD. Researchers looking at OCD have used a scale called the Yale-Brown Obsessive-Compulsive Scale, or Y-BOCS. Dr. Phillips has developed a modification of this scale for BDD and logically called it the BDD-YBOCS. We present it here to help you further measure the severity of your body-image problem.

The BDD-YBOCS is derived from the Y-BOCS, which is used to assess severity of OCD. We have included the BDD-YBOCS here in the form below, developed by Phillips and her colleagues in 1997 and recently revised. This scale was designed for use by clinicians interviewing patients with BDD. Just below the heading we have changed the phrase "the patient" to "your experience," but none of the other wording has been changed. The BDD-YBOCS was developed to be used by a mental health professional, who would ask the questions of the patient. We are using it here as a self-report scale. Since no research has been done on the use of it as a self-report measure we recommend that you interpret your score with caution. On item 11, please ignore the instructions that refer to the BABS questions. Also please remember that although this scale is used in the book with permission of the author, it is copyrighted and as a result may not be copied or distributed further without the author's permission.

The BDD-YBOCS*

For each item circle the number identifying the response which best characterizes your experience during the **past week.**

1. *Time occupied* by thoughts about body defect
   How much of your time is occupied by THOUGHTS about a defect or flaw in your appearance [list body parts of concern]?

   0 = None
   1 = Mild (less than 1 hr/day)
   2 = Moderate (1–3 hrs/day)
   3 = Severe (greater than 3 and up to 8 hrs/day)
   4 = Extreme (greater than 8 hrs/day)

2. *Interference* due to thoughts about body defect
   How much do your THOUGHTS about your body defect(s) interfere with your social or work (role) functioning? (Is there anything you aren't doing or can't do because of them?)

   Y/N Spending time with friends
   Y/N Dating
   Y/N Attending social functions
   Y/N Doing things with family in and outside of home
   Y/N Going to school/work each day
   Y/N Being on time for or missing school/work
   Y/N Focusing at school/work
   Y/N Productivity at school/work
   Y/N Doing homework or maintaining grades
   Y/N Daily activities

   0 = None
   1 = Mild, slight interference with social, occupational, or role activities, but overall performance not impaired.
   2 = Moderate, definite interference with social, occupational, or role performance, but still manageable.
   3 = Severe, causes substantial impairment of social, occupational, or role performance.
   4 = Extreme, incapacitating.

3. *Distress* associated with thoughts about body defect
   How much distress do your THOUGHTS about your body defect(s) cause you? *Rate "disturbing" feelings or anxiety that seem to be triggered by these thoughts, not general anxiety or anxiety associated with other symptoms.*

   0 = None
   1 = Mild, not too disturbing.
   2 = Moderate, disturbing.
   3 = Severe, very disturbing.
   4 = Extreme, disabling distress.

* The BDD-YBOCS, from article by Phillips, Hollander, Rasmussen, Aronowitz, DeCaria, and Goodman (1997). Reprinted with permission from authors.

For each item circle the number identifying the response which best characterizes your experience during the past week.

4. Resistance against thoughts of body defect
   How much of an effort do you make to resist these THOUGHTS? [*Pause*] How often do you try to disregard them or turn your attention away from these thoughts as they enter your mind?
   Only rate effort made to resist, NOT success or failure in actually controlling the thoughts. How much patient resists the thoughts may or may not correlate with ability to control them.

   0 = Makes an effort to always resist, or symptoms so minimal doesn't need to actively resist.
   1 = Tries to resist most of time.
   2 = Makes some effort to resist.
   3 = Yields to all such thoughts without attempting to control them but yields with some reluctance.
   4 = Completely and willingly yields to all such thoughts.

5. *Degree of control* over thoughts about body defect
   How much control do you have over your THOUGHTS about your body defect(s)? How successful are you in stopping or diverting these thoughts?

   0 = Complete control, or no need for control because thoughts are so minimal.
   1 = Much control, usually able to stop or divert these thoughts with some effort and concentration.
   2 = Moderate control, sometimes able to stop or divert these thoughts.
   3 = Little control, rarely successful in stopping thoughts, can only divert attention with difficulty.
   4 = No control, experienced as completely involuntary, rarely able to even momentarily divert attention.

6. *Time spent* in activities related to body defect
   The next several questions are about the activities/behaviors you do in relation to your body defects.

   0 = None
   1 = Mild (spends less than 1 hr/day)
   2 = Moderate (1–3 hrs/day)
   3 = Severe (spends more than 3 and up to 8 hours/day)
   4 = Extreme (spends more than 8 hrs/day in these activities)

   Read list of activities below to determine which ones the patient engages in.
   How much time do you spend in ACTIVITIES related to your concern over your appearance [read activities patient engages in]?

   Read list of activities (check all that apply)

   ____ Checking mirrors/other surfaces

   ____ Grooming activities

   ____ Applying makeup

   ____ Excessive exercise (time beyond 1 hr. a day)

_____ Camouflaging with clothing/other cover (rate time spent selecting/changing clothes, not time wearing them)

_____ Scrutinizing others' appearance (comparing)

_____ Questioning others about/discussing your appearance

_____ Picking at skin

_____ Other

For each item circle the number identifying the response which best characterizes your experience during the past week.

7. _Interference_ due to activities related to body defect
How much do these ACTIVITIES interfere with your social or work (role) functioning? (Is there anything you don't do because of them?)

0 = None
1 = Mild, slight interference with social, occupational, or role activities, but overall performance not impaired.
2 = Moderate, definite interference with social, occupational, or role performance, but still manageable.
3 = Severe, causes substantial impairment in social, occupational, or role performance.
4 = Extreme, incapacitating.

8. _Distress_ associated with activities related to body defect
How would you feel if you were prevented from performing these ACTIVITIES? How anxious would you become?
Rate degree of distress/frustration patient would experience if performance of the activities was suddenly interrupted.

0 = None
1 = Mild, only slightly anxious if behavior prevented.
2 = Moderate, reports that anxiety would mount but remain manageable if behavior is prevented.
3 = Severe, prominent and very disturbing increase in anxiety if behavior is interrupted.
4 = Extreme, incapacitating anxiety from any intervention aimed at modifying activity.

9. Res_istance_ against compulsions
How much of an effort do you make to resist these ACTIVITIES?
Only rate effort made to resist, NOT success or failure in actually controlling the activities. How much the patient resists these behaviors may or may not correlate with his/her ability to control them.

0 = Makes an effort to always resist, or symptoms so minimal doesn't need to actively resist.
1 = Tries to resist most of the time.
2 = Makes some effort to resist.
3 = Yields to almost all of these behaviors without attempting to control them, but does so with some reluctance.
4 = Completely and willingly yields to all behaviors related to body defect.

For each item circle the number identifying the response which best characterizes your experience during the past week.

10. *Degree of control* over compulsive behavior
    How strong is the drive to perform these behaviors? How much control do you have over them?

    0 = Complete control, or control is unnecessary because symptoms are mild.
    1 = Much control, experiences pressure to perform the behavior, but usually able to exercise voluntary control over it.
    2 = Moderate control, strong pressure to perform behavior, can control it only with difficulty.
    3 = Little control, very strong drive to perform behavior, must be carried to completion, can delay only with difficulty.
    4 = No control, drive to perform behavior experienced as completely involuntary and overpowering, rarely able to even momentarily delay activity.

11. *Insight*
    This question should not be asked to the patient. Instead, complete the BABS, and then return to this question afterwards and score it based on the responses to the BABS questions.
    Is it possible that your defect might be less noticeable or less unattractive than you think it is? [*Pause*] How convinced are you that [fill in body part] is as unattractive as you think it is? [*Pause*] Can anyone convince you that it doesn't look so bad?

    0 = Excellent insight, fully rational.
    1 = Good insight. Readily acknowledges absurdity of thoughts (but doesn't seem completely convinced that there isn't something besides anxiety to be concerned about).
    2 = Fair insight. Reluctantly admits that thoughts seem unreasonable but wavers.
    3 = Poor insight. Maintains that thoughts are not unreasonable.
    4 = Lacks insight, delusional. Definitely convinced that concerns are reasonable, unresponsive to contrary evidence.

12. *Avoidance*
    Have you been avoiding doing anything, going any place, or being with anyone because of your thoughts or behaviors related to your body defects? *If YES, then ask*: What do you avoid?
    Rate degree to which patient deliberately tries to avoid things such as social interactions or work-related activities. Do not include avoidance of mirrors or avoidance of compulsive behaviors.

    0 = No deliberate avoidance.
    1 = Mild, minimal avoidance.
    2 = Moderate, some avoidance clearly present.
    3 = Severe, much avoidance; avoidance prominent.
    4 = Extreme, very extensive avoidance; patient avoids almost all activities.

Brackets [ ] indicate material that should be read. Brackets are also used to indicate a pause.

Parentheses ( ) indicate optional material that may be read.

Italicized items are instructions to the interviewer.

Instructions for the BDD-YBOCS (8/97)

Purpose: This rating scale is designed to rate the severity and type of symptoms in patients with body dysmorphic disorder (BDD). BDD is defined as a preoccupation with an imagined or slight defect in appearance—for example, "thinning" hair, a "large" nose, or a "scarred" face. The scale is derived from the Yale-Brown Obsessive Compulsive Scale (Y-BOCS). Like the Y-BOCS, the first 5 items rate BDD-related *preoccupations*, and the second 5 items rate BDD-related *behaviors*. The BDD-YBOCS also rates *insight* (item 11) and *avoidance* (item 12).

Format: This rating scale is intended for use as a semi-structured interview. The interviewer should assess the items in the listed order and read the questions provided. However, the interviewer is free to ask additional questions for purposes of clarification. In general, the ratings should depend on the patient's report; however, the final rating is based on the interviewer's clinical judgment.

- Brackets [ ] indicate material that should be read. Brackets are also used to indicate a pause.

- Parentheses ( ) indicate optional material that may be read.

- Italicized items are instructions to the interviewer.

Sources of Information: If the patient volunteers information at any time during the interview, that information should be considered. Ratings should be based primarily on reports and observations gained during the interview. Additional information supplied by others (e.g., spouse or parent) may be included in a determination of the ratings only if it is judged that 1) such information is essential to adequately assessing symptom severity, *and* 2) consistent week-to-week reporting can be ensured by having the same informant(s) present for each rating session. If you judge that the information being provided is grossly inaccurate, then the reliability of the patient or informant is in doubt and should be noted accordingly on the interview.

Ratings: Rate each item *during the past week* up until and including the time of the interview. Scores should reflect the average (mean) occurrence of each item for the entire week. For questions 1 through 5 (which rate BDD-related preoccupations), rate the *total* (composite) effect of *all* body parts of concern. For items 6 through 10 (which rate BDD-related behaviors), also rate the *total* (composite) effect of *all* behaviors. For items 9 and 10 (resistance and control items), if the patient's responses differ for different behaviors, select the response that represents an average score for the different behaviors. For item 12, do not rate avoidance of compulsive behaviors such as looking at mirrors; instead, rate the extent to which the patient avoids activities that contribute to adequate functioning—e.g., avoidance of social interactions or work-related activities.

Diagnosing BDD: Before proceeding with questions 1–5, you must first determine that the patient has BDD and identify the body parts with which he or she is excessively concerned. The diagnosis is made if the person is preoccupied with an imagined defect in appearance; if a slight physical anomaly is present, the person's concern must be markedly excessive. Any body part can be the focus of concern, and patients are commonly preoccupied with more than one body part. In addition, the preoccupation must have caused clinically significant distress or impairment in social, occupational, or other important areas of functioning. Finally, to receive a diagnosis of BDD the preoccupation cannot be better accounted for by another mental disorder (for example, the person's concern cannot be limited to body shape and size if he or she has anorexia nervosa). It is important that only those concerns related to ugliness or a sense of physical defectiveness be rated. For example, if a patient dislikes his self-inflicted wounds because they remind him that he is mentally ill, do not rate this concern with the BDD-YBOCS.

To determine whether the person has BDD, and to identify the body parts of concern, the following questions should be asked:

"Are you very worried about your appearance in any way?"

IF YES: What is your concern? Do you think [body part] is especially unattractive? What about the appearance of your face, skin, hair, nose, or the shape/size/other aspect of any other part of your body? _____

_____

"Does this concern preoccupy you? That is, you think about it a lot, and wish you could worry about it less? Do others say you're more concerned about [body part] than you should be?" _____

_____

_____

"What effect does this preoccupation have on your life? Does it cause you a lot of distress? Does your concern have any effect on your family or friends?"_____

_____

_____

List body parts of concern here: _____

_____

_____

Identifying BDD Behaviors: Associated behaviors, which are inquired about with questions 6 through 10, must also be identified before proceeding with the interview. They can be identified by asking the patient whether he/she engages in any behaviors in association with his/her concern about the "defect." The following behaviors, which are common in BDD, should be specifically asked about (*check all that apply*):

_____ Checking the "defect" in mirrors or other reflecting surfaces (or checking it directly if visible without the use of a mirror)

_____ Seeking reassurance from others about the appearance of the body part

_____ Asking others to look at or verify the existence of the "deformity"

_____ Requests for surgery, dermatologic treatment, or other treatment

_____ Comparison of the body part with the same body part of others

_____ Touching the body part

_____ Grooming behaviors (for example, hair combing, hair styling, or shaving)

_____ Skin picking

_____ Applying makeup

_____ Camouflaging (for example, with makeup or with hats or other clothing)

_____ Rearranging clothing to hide the "defect"

_____ Other; describe: _____

On repeated testing, you should review and, if necessary, revise the list of "defects" and associated behaviors before doing the ratings. It is useful to be aware of past symptoms because they may re-appear during subsequent testing.

Lilly's Answers to The BDD-YBOCS*

For each item circle the number identifying the response which best characterizes your experience during the **past week.**

1. *Time occupied* by thoughts about body defect
   How much of your time is occupied by THOUGHTS about a defect or flaw in your appearance [list body parts of concern]?

   0 = None
   1 = Mild (less than 1 hr/day)
   2 = Moderate (1–3 hrs/day)
   (3)= Severe (greater than 3 and up to 8 hrs/day)
   4 = Extreme (greater than 8 hrs/day)

2. *Interference* due to thoughts about body defect
   How much do your THOUGHTS about your body defect(s) interfere with your social or work (role) functioning? (Is there anything you aren't doing or can't do because of them?)

   0 = None
   1 = Mild, slight interference with social, occupational, or role activities, but overall performance not impaired.
   (2)= Moderate, definite interference with social, occupational, or role performance, but still manageable.
   3 = Severe, causes substantial impairment of social, occupational, or role performance.
   4 = Extreme, incapacitating.

3. *Distress* associated with thoughts about body defect
   How much distress do your THOUGHTS about your body defect(s) cause you? *Rate "disturbing" feelings or anxiety that seem to be triggered by these thoughts, not general anxiety or anxiety associated with other symptoms.*

   0 = None
   1 = Mild, not too disturbing.

$\bigcirc{2}$ = Moderate, disturbing.
3 = Severe, very disturbing.
4 = Extreme, disabling distress.

4. Resistance against thoughts of body defect
How much of an effort do you make to resist these THOUGHTS? [*Pause*] How often do you try to disregard them or turn your attention away from these thoughts as they enter your mind?
Only rate effort made to resist, NOT success or failure in actually controlling the thoughts. How much patient resists the thoughts may or may not correlate with ability to control them.

0 = Makes an effort to always resist, or symptoms so minimal doesn't need to actively resist.
$\bigcirc{1}$ = Tries to resist most of time.
2 = Makes some effort to resist.
3 = Yields to all such thoughts without attempting to control them but yields with some reluctance.
4 = Completely and willingly yields to all such thoughts.

For each item circle the number identifying the response which best characterizes your experience during the past week.

5. *Degree of control* over thoughts about body defect
How much control do you have over your THOUGHTS about your body defect(s)? How successful are you in stopping or diverting these thoughts?

0 = Complete control, or no need for control because thoughts are so minimal.
1 = Much control, usually able to stop or divert these thoughts with some effort and concentration.
$\bigcirc{2}$ = Moderate control, sometimes able to stop or divert these thoughts.
3 = Little control, rarely successful in stopping thoughts, can only divert attention with difficulty.
4 = No control, experienced as completely involuntary, rarely able to even momentarily divert attention.

6. *Time spent* in activities related to body defect
The next several questions are about the activities/behaviors you do in relation to your body defects.

0 = None
1 = Mild (spends less than 1 hr/day)
2 = Moderate (1–3 hrs/day)
$\bigcirc{3}$ = Severe (spends more than 3 and up to 8 hours/day)
4 = Extreme (spends more than 8 hrs/day in these activities)

Read list of activities below to determine which ones the patient engages in.
How much time do you spend in ACTIVITIES related to your concern over your appearance [read activities patient engages in]?

Read list of activities (check all that apply)
___✓ Checking mirrors/other surfaces
___✓ Grooming activities

_____ Applying makeup

__✓ Excessive exercise (time beyond 1 hr. a day)

__✓ Camouflaging with clothing/other cover (rate time spent selecting/changing clothes, not time wearing them)

__✓ Scrutinizing others' appearance (comparing)

__✓ Questioning others about/discussing your appearance

_____ Picking at skin

_____ Other

7. *Interference* due to activities related to body defect

How much do these ACTIVITIES interfere with your social or work (role) functioning? (Is there anything you don't do because of them?)

0 = None

1 = Mild, slight interference with social, occupational, or role activities, but overall performance not impaired.

(2) = Moderate, definite interference with social, occupational, or role performance, but still manageable.

3 = Severe, causes substantial impairment in social, occupational, or role performance.

4 = Extreme, incapacitating.

8. *Distress* associated with activities related to body defect

How would you feel if you were prevented from performing these ACTIVITIES? How anxious would you become?

Rate degree of distress/frustration patient would experience if performance of the activities was suddenly interrupted.

0 = None

1 = Mild, only slightly anxious if behavior prevented.

(2) = Moderate, reports that anxiety would mount but remain manageable if behavior is prevented.

3 = Severe, prominent and very disturbing increase in anxiety if behavior is interrupted.

4 = Extreme, incapacitating anxiety from any intervention aimed at modifying activity.

9. Re*sistance* against compulsions

How much of an effort do you make to resist these ACTIVITIES?

Only rate effort made to resist, NOT success or failure in actually controlling the activities. How much the patient resists these behaviors may or may not correlate with his/her ability to control them.

0 = Makes an effort to always resist, or symptoms so minimal doesn't need to actively resist.

(1) = Tries to resist most of the time.

2 = Makes some effort to resist.

3 = Yields to almost all of these behaviors without attempting to control them, but does so with some reluctance.

4 = Completely and willingly yields to all behaviors related to body defect.

10. *Degree of control* over compulsive behavior

How strong is the drive to perform these behaviors? How much control do you have over them?

0 = Complete control, or control is unnecessary because symptoms are mild.

1 = Much control, experiences pressure to perform the behavior, but usually able to exercise voluntary control over it.

(2)= Moderate control, strong pressure to perform behavior, can control it only with difficulty.

3 = Little control, very strong drive to perform behavior, must be carried to completion, can delay only with difficulty.

4 = No control, drive to perform behavior experienced as completely involuntary and overpowering, rarely able to even momentarily delay activity.

For each item circle the number identifying the response which best characterizes your experience during the past week.

11. *Insight*

This question should not be asked to the patient. Instead, complete the BABS, and then return to this question afterwards and score it based on the responses to the BABS questions.

Is it possible that your defect might be less noticeable or less unattractive than you think it is? [*Pause*] How convinced are you that [fill in body part] is as unattractive as you think it is? [*Pause*] Can anyone convince you that it doesn't look so bad?

0 = Excellent insight, fully rational.

1 = Good insight. Readily acknowledges absurdity of thoughts (but doesn't seem completely convinced that there isn't something besides anxiety to be concerned about).

(2)= Fair insight. Reluctantly admits that thoughts seem unreasonable but wavers.

3 = Poor insight. Maintains that thoughts are not unreasonable.

4 = Lacks insight, delusional. Definitely convinced that concerns are reasonable, unresponsive to contrary evidence.

12. *Avoidance*

Have you been avoiding doing anything, going any place, or being with anyone because of your thoughts or behaviors related to your body defects? *If YES, then ask:* What do you avoid?

Rate degree to which patient deliberately tries to avoid things such as social interactions or work-related activities. Do not include avoidance of mirrors or avoidance of compulsive behaviors.

0 = No deliberate avoidance.

1 = Mild, minimal avoidance.

2 = Moderate, some avoidance clearly present.

(3)= Severe, much avoidance; avoidance prominent.

4 = Extreme, very extensive avoidance; patient avoids almost all activities.

Brackets [ ] indicate material that should be read. Brackets are also used to indicate a pause.

Parentheses ( ) indicate optional material that may be read.

Italicized items are instructions to the interviewer.

Instructions for the BDD-YBOCS (8/97)

Purpose: This rating scale is designed to rate the severity and type of symptoms in patients with body dysmorphic disorder (BDD). BDD is defined as a preoccupation with an imagined or slight defect in appearance—for example, "thinning" hair, a "large" nose, or a "scarred" face. The scale is derived from the Yale-Brown Obsessive Compulsive Scale (Y-BOCS). Like the Y-BOCS, the first 5 items rate BDD-related*preoccupations*, and the second 5 items rate BDD-related *behaviors*. The BDD-YBOCS also rates *insight* (item 11) and *avoidance* (item 12).

Format: This rating scale is intended for use as a semi-structured interview. The interviewer should assess the items in the listed order and read the questions provided. However, the interviewer is free to ask additional questions for purposes of clarification. In general, the ratings should depend on the patient's report; however, the final rating is based on the interviewer's clinical judgment.

- Brackets [ ] indicate material that should be read. Brackets are also used to indicate a pause.

- Parentheses ( ) indicate optional material that may be read.

- Italicized items are instructions to the interviewer.

Sources of Information: If the patient volunteers information at any time during the interview, that information should be considered. Ratings should be based primarily on reports and observations gained during the interview. Additional information supplied by others (e.g., spouse or parent) may be included in a determination of the ratings only if it is judged that 1) such information is essential to adequately assessing symptom severity, *and* 2) consistent week-to-week reporting can be ensured by having the same informant(s) present for each rating session. If you judge that the information being provided is grossly inaccurate, then the reliability of the patient or informant is in doubt and should be noted accordingly on the interview.

Ratings: Rate each item *during the past week* up until and including the time of the interview. Scores should reflect the average (mean) occurrence of each item for the entire week. For questions 1 through 5 (which rate BDD-related preoccupations), rate the *total* (composite) effect of *all* body parts of concern. For items 6 through 10 (which rate BDD-related behaviors), also rate the *total* (composite) effect of *all* behaviors. For items 9 and 10 (resistance and control items), if the patient's responses differ for different behaviors, select the response that represents an average score for the different behaviors. For item 12, do not rate avoidance of compulsive behaviors such as looking at mirrors; instead, rate the extent to which the patient avoids activities that contribute to adequate functioning—e.g., avoidance of social interactions or work-related activities.

Diagnosing BDD: Before proceeding with questions 1–5, you must first determine that the patient has BDD and identify the body parts with which he or she is excessively concerned. The diagnosis is made if the person is preoccupied with an imagined defect in appearance; if a slight physical anomaly is present, the person's concern must be markedly excessive. Any body part can be the focus of concern, and patients are commonly preoccupied with more than one body part. In addition, the preoccupation must have caused clinically significant distress or impairment in social, occupational, or other important areas of functioning. Finally, to receive a diagnosis of BDD the preoccupation cannot be better accounted for by another mental disorder (for example, the person's concern cannot be limited to body shape and size if he or she has anorexia nervosa). It is important that only those concerns related to ugliness or a sense of physical defectiveness be rated. For example, if a patient dislikes his self-inflicted wounds because they remind him that he is mentally ill, do not rate this concern with the BDD-YBOCS.

To determine whether the person has BDD, and to identify the body parts of concern, the following questions should be asked:

Are you very worried about your appearance in any way? _Yes_____

IF YES: What is your concern? Do you think [body part] is especially unattractive? What about the appearance of your face, skin, hair, nose, or the shape/size/other aspect of any other part of your body? _I think my stomach and thighs are huge. I'm fairly satisfied with the rest of my body._

Does this concern preoccupy you? That is, you think about it a lot, and wish you could worry about it less? Do others say you're more concerned about [body part] than you should be? _I think about it all the time. My husband says I worry too much about it and doesn't understand why I am so very concerned about the size and looks of my stomach and thighs. I wish I could stop thinking about it, but I just can't seem to be able to stop the thoughts._

What effect does this preoccupation have on your life? Does it cause you a lot of distress? Does your concern have any effect on your family or friends? _This preoccupation is ruining my life. I hate to go out and when I do I worry about how I look. My husband is having trouble understanding, and I'm short-tempered and impatient with my kids._

List body parts of concern here: _Stomach, thighs_____

Identifying BDD Behaviors: Associated behaviors, which are inquired about with questions 6 through 10, must also be identified before proceeding with the interview. They can be identified by asking the patient whether he/she engages in any behaviors in association with his/her concern about the "defect." The following behaviors, which are common in BDD, should be specifically asked about (check all that apply):

_x_ Checking the "defect" in mirrors or other reflecting surfaces (or checking it directly if visible without the use of a mirror)

_x_ Seeking reassurance from others about the appearance of the body part

_x_ Asking others to look at or verify the existence of the "deformity"

____ Requests for surgery, dermatologic treatment, or other treatment

_x_ Comparison of the body part with the same body part of others

_x_ Touching the body part

____ Grooming behaviors (for example, hair combing, hair styling, or shaving)

____ Skin picking

____ Applying makeup

_x_ Camouflaging (for example, with makeup or with hats or other clothing) __x__ Rearranging clothing to hide the "defect"

_____ Other; describe:_____

On repeated testing, you should review and, if necessary, revise the list of "defects" and associated behaviors before doing the ratings. It is useful to be aware of past symptoms because they may re-appear during subsequent testing.

Scoring the BDD-YBOCS

If, after reviewing the BDDE-SR earlier in this chapter, you believe you have BDD, then read on about how to interpret your BDD-YBOCS score. If you believe you have another disorder that is associated with body-image problems, such as anorexia nervosa, you can use this scale to see how severe your body-image concerns are.

If you scored between 0 and 9, either you don't have BDD, or it is extremely mild. Some people will end up with scores in this range after treatment. A score of 10 to 15 shows BDD that is mild but probably worth treating. People who score in this range may do well with therapy alone or by working through this book by themselves. If you scored between 16 and 25 you likely have moderately severe BDD. Most people who score in this range can probably get some help from this book but would be wise to see a therapist familiar with BDD and related disorders, such as OCD. You may want to consider taking medication, especially if you are also depressed. If your score is 26 or higher you probably have severe BDD. We strongly recommend that you get professional help from someone knowledgeable about BDD. You are likely to need both medication and therapy. Show this book to your therapist and let him or her review your answers to the questions in this chapter.

Lilly's score was 25, which indicates that she probably had moderately severe BDD. Medication and cognitive behavioral therapy with a therapist were appropriate options for her. Medication helped her deal with her depression and anxiety while she was learning the cognitive behavioral skills needed to bring her body image into better balance.

In the next chapter we will further explain the treatment of BDD and body-image concerns, including the role of medications. In the Balanced Image Program, you will be guided through the understanding of BDD and its treatment. You may choose to work through the program on your own, or with the assistance of a therapist who treats BDD.

CHAPTER 5

The Treatment of BDD

Research on body dysmorphic disorder is in its infancy. So far, two methods for treating BDD have been identified as helpful. Medication is often used to help relieve depression and obsessive thoughts. Cognitive behavioral therapy (CBT), which is used in the Balanced Image Program described here, is the other treatment helpful for body-image dissatisfaction and body dysmorphic disorder.

The Balanced Image Program has five goals:

- to help you bring your body image perception into balance,

- to help you develop a healthier response to your body image,

- to help you develop a more balanced *ideal* body image based less on cultural influence and peer pressure,

- to help you develop a healthy response to discrepancies between your ideal body image and your actual body image, and

- to help you find new ways of defining yourself and discover other aspects of self-image and self-esteem.

We'll meet these goals by drawing on the knowledge and research of experts in several areas. Since balancing body image involves change, we'll begin by exploring the latest information about how and why people change. Body image is only a part of overall self-image; we'll help you examine other parts of your self-image and enhance your self-image and self-esteem by guiding you to balance your emphasis on the various components of your self-image. We'll also help you learn to recognize the abundant messages in our culture about appearance, and your automatic responses to them, and develop a healthier response.

The core of the program is cognitive behavioral therapy. This therapy method involves changing thought patterns and behavior. Let's take a closer look at the roots of this type of therapy and how it can assist us in making changes in our perception of and response to our body image.

Behavior Therapy

Behavior therapy and *behavior modification* are terms that refer to the application of knowledge about how people learn and change to helping people who have behaviors or disorders that interfere with their life. The emphasis is on changing specific problem behaviors, not on changing a person's personality or making them become a different person. Slightly different meanings and some different traditions are connected to the terms, which are most likely to interest historians or psychologists. For our purposes, we could use the terms interchangeably. The methods used in behavior therapy begin with the identification of the problem or target behavior. It is often useful to think about behaviors as excesses or deficits. A *behavioral excess* is a behavior you do too much, too often, or for too long. On the other hand, a *behavioral deficit* is one that you do too infrequently, too little, or for too little time.

Behavior therapy traces its roots to work on learning in the early to mid-twentieth century, including Ivan Pavlov and his study of learned behavior in dogs, and B. F. Skinner and his work with animals and people. Skinner studied how reinforcement works, and his ideas have been translated into principles applied in areas ranging from schools to therapy. Scientists have developed the ideas first learned in the animal laboratory, refining them and expanding on them to help people with behavior change.

One particular technique, *exposure and response prevention* (ERP), has been used for many years to treat obsessive-compulsive disorder. In chapter 1, we discussed how BDD and OCD are sometimes thought to be on the same spectrum of related disorders. ERP has also been proven to be effective in reducing the obsessions and compulsions involved in BDD. Even if you don't have BDD or obsessions and compulsions, ERP will be an important part of your Balanced Image Program. Exposure and response prevention will help you change the way you deal with body-image concerns and reduce the excessive behaviors associated with these concerns.

What exactly is ERP? *Exposure* involves placing yourself in situations that cause worry, distress, disgust, or anxiety. Repeated exposure, without your usual response to relieve or avoid your distress, will help you realize that the feared negative consequences don't occur or aren't as bad as you thought they would be. In other words, your negative reaction fades. At first, these exposures will be upsetting or anxiety provoking, but with repeated exposure the distress will be reduced. This process is called *habituation*. It sounds hard, doesn't it? If you started with the most upsetting situation, it would probably be overwhelming, but we will help you rank situations on a hierarchy, from the most upsetting to the least upsetting. We will recommend that you start exposure with a situation in the middle, one you feel you can handle even though it is upsetting, then proceed to situations higher up on your hierarchy.

Response prevention involves discontinuing behaviors you use to make yourself feel better about your body image. Sometimes this will mean stopping a particular behavior altogether, but more often it will mean reducing the frequency of the behavior, spending less time on it, or changing the way you do it. For example, you might spend fifteen minutes styling your hair instead of an hour. Then you might check your hair in the bathroom mirror only at lunchtime instead of every half hour. Again, you will make a hierarchy of behaviors according to how distressing it would be to give them up, and begin with response prevention for a behavior midway up on the hierarchy.

Nathan Azrin and Gregory Nunn (1977) developed a behavior modification procedure, called *habit reversal*, that can be applied to unwanted habits and behavior disorders. We will use habit reversal techniques to help you change some of your habitual behaviors associated with body-image dissatisfaction. This will be especially helpful for people who engage in excessive grooming activities or skin picking, common problems among people with BDD.

Cognitive Therapy

Aaron T. Beck, M.D., developed *cognitive therapy* in the 1960s. It began as a short-term treatment for depression that focused on solving current problems and modifying dysfunctional thinking and behavior. Since then, Beck and others have adapted cognitive therapy to treat other problems, including body dysmorphic disorder, generalized anxiety disorder, panic disorder, social phobia, substance abuse, eating disorders, obsessive-compulsive disorder, post-traumatic stress disorder, personality disorders, chronic pain, hypochondriasis, and schizophrenia (Beck 1995). Since the 1960s, numerous researchers have added to Aaron Beck's work. Several variations on cognitive therapy have been developed, including rational emotive therapy (RET), which was developed by Albert

Ellis. An important part of developing a balanced self-image is learning to think about yourself differently. This book will show you how to use the methods developed in cognitive therapy to help you change the way you think.

Cognitive Behavioral Therapy

In recent years most clinicians working with cognitive therapy or behavior therapy have started to call what they do *cognitive behavioral therapy*. This is because they combine traditional ideas from behavior therapy and newer ideas from cognitive therapy to develop the most effective treatments. The cognitive aspect of this type of therapy is focused on how we think and how that relates to the way we feel and behave. Much of the thinking we do is in the form of self-talk. Until now, your self-talk has contributed to or served to maintain your problem with self-image. However, just as self-talk can be harmful, it can also help you develop a more balanced response to your body image. *The BDD Workbook* will help you make changes in your perception of and response to your body image by combining behavioral change methods, such as ERP and habit reversal, with cognitive methods, such as keeping track of and changing self-talk.

Medication

People with diagnosable BDD may get significant help from certain medications. The group of medications known as serotonin reuptake inhibitors (SRIs) that are effective in the treatment of obsessive-compulsive disorder (OCD) is often effective in treating BDD. These include citalopram (Celexa), clomipramine (Anafranil), fluoxetine (Prozac), fluvoxamine (Luvox), paroxetine (Paxil), sertraline (Zoloft), and possibly venlafaxine (Effexor). Serotonin reuptake inhibitors are classified as antidepressants, but could also be called anti-obsessionals because they often reduce obsessions in people with OCD and BDD. When the obsessions are reduced, people have less drive to perform their compulsions. These medications work by changing the way serotonin is handled in the brain. Serotonin is necessary for the communication between nerve cells in the brain.

Your doctor may prescribe one of these medications. If you try taking an SRI and it doesn't help relieve BDD symptoms, don't give up: it may take up to twelve weeks or longer after reaching a high dosage to get results, and all SRIs don't help everyone. Sometimes one doesn't help a particular patient and a different SRI must be tried. If several SRIs are tried and found ineffective, other medications can be added to help achieve a therapeutic response. People with this disorder will want to discuss medications with their doctor. This is especially important for those with serious depression and suicidal thoughts, which are often part of the picture in BDD. The SRI will usually ease both the depression and BDD symptoms. Most people with severe BDD symptoms and those with poor insight (they *really* believe their obsessive thoughts) should consider taking medication, even if they are not depressed. Medication can relieve BDD and depression symptoms enough to make cognitive behavioral therapy possible. Starting on medication doesn't mean a lifelong commitment. You could use it while you are doing CBT, then after you are feeling better, consult your doctor about reducing or stopping the medication. At this point no studies have been done that show CBT prevents relapse of BDD after medication has stopped. Research on treatment of other disorders such as depression with cognitive behavioral therapy has shown a reduction in the rate of relapse in people who were taught mindfulness meditation and treated with therapy.

What Usually Does Not Work

Many people with BDD seek nonpsychiatric medical or surgical treatment for their perceived defect. Because the perceived defect is minimal or nonexistent, many are turned down for cosmetic surgery. They may go from surgeon to surgeon until they finally get someone to perform the surgery. While most people without BDD are satisfied with the results of cosmetic surgeries, researcher Katharine Phillips has found that about two-thirds of BDD patients who undergo cosmetic surgery experience no change in, or a worsening of, their concerns after surgery. Preoccupation with and distress about the perceived defect remains the same or worsens (Phillips 1996). Researchers estimate that about 7 percent of women and perhaps a third of men seeking cosmetic surgery are suffering from BDD (Pope, Phillips, and Olivardia 2000).

For example, Cameron felt that one side of his jaw was much larger than the other side. There actually was some asymmetry in Cameron's jaw, so a doctor agreed to perform surgery. Cameron was happy with the results at first, but he continued to check his jaw in the mirror. He even bought a tape measure and measured each side of his face. He looked at other people's jaws to see if he could detect any asymmetry. To him, the asymmetry in his jaw always seemed much worse than anyone else's. Cameron consulted several surgeons and had surgery again. Twice more! Still, after three surgeries on his jaw, he felt that his face looked worse than ever, and he even considered suicide.

Gradually, Cameron accepted his "deformed" jaw, but he began to notice that his nose was much too long and "bumpy." He sought a new surgeon to perform surgery on his nose. After consulting three surgeons, he found one who agreed to perform a rhinoplasty (cosmetic surgery on the nose). Again, Cameron was happy at first, but he soon was back in the surgeon's office, demanding a correction. Cameron broke down in the office. In tears, he told the doctor about the surgeries on his jaw. He threatened to commit suicide if the doctor couldn't make his nose look right. The surgeon referred Cameron to a psychiatrist, and as a result he was successfully treated with cognitive behavioral therapy and medication. Today, Cameron is still unsatisfied with his nose and his jaw, but it doesn't seem as important to him. He has decided to accept his face as it is. As you can see, cosmetic surgery isn't an effective treatment for people with BDD.

What about hypnosis, natural remedies, or diets? There is no evidence that hypnosis, herbs, supplements, or diets can significantly reduce the obsessive thoughts and compulsive behaviors of BDD or related disorders, such as OCD. What about psychotherapy, including uncovering childhood trauma? This type of treatment may help reduce other psychological symptoms, but used alone it is not sufficient treatment for BDD.

Many people with muscle dysmorphia or with obsessions about weight may try diet supplements, diet pills, extreme diets to lose or gain weight, or even anabolic steroids, believing that gaining a few more pounds of muscle or losing a few pounds of fat might help. This approach almost never works. The person usually finds that a few more pounds aren't enough, which leads him or her to try more supplements, stricter diets, extensive workout routines, or more steroids. If BDD is the problem, efforts to improve body appearance will not be helpful.

When to Seek Further Help

If your answers to the questions in chapter 4 suggest you have BDD, we advise you to consult a psychiatrist or psychologist. You will want to look for one who knows about BDD and related disorders like OCD. He or she can give you an accurate diagnosis and help you decide on a course of treatment. If you can't find someone who has expertise in these types of problems, a seasoned therapist with limited BDD experience could use *The BDD Workbook* as a guide to coach you through the Balanced Image Program. If you choose to use *The BDD Workbook* by yourself and you find that it seems too difficult or you are very depressed—and especially if you have suicidal thoughts—you need to seek professional help immediately.

Change is not easy, but having knowledge can ease the process. Change may seem unattainable now, but knowledge and application of cognitive behavioral therapy can bring about success. Understanding the process of change is an important part of cognitive behavioral therapy and the changing process itself. Understanding helps relieve some of the fears and doubts that are inevitably linked to change. Chapter 6 will help you recognize these fears and doubts and then examine, confront, and deal with them. By the end of the chapter, you will have made a decision: to change the way you view and respond to your body image, or to remain the same.

While you are considering that decision, we have homework for you to do. The Self-Image Journal will help you keep track of your feelings, thoughts, and behaviors concerning body image and self-image. Make copies of the blank Self-Image Journal and start a new one each day. You will continue to keep the journal as you work through the Balanced Image Program. The information you gather in your journal will be used in many of the exercises. There are no right or wrong answers. Record any situation that challenges your self-image. The situations can be as simple as looking in the mirror and having negative thoughts about how you look, or as complex as measuring the reactions of others at a party. We have included Lilly's Self-Image Journal from her first days of the Balanced Image Program as an example. As you continue through the program, we will give you instructions to include more specific information in your journal.

Self-Image Journal

Date: _____

Challenging Situation	Response		
	Behavior and Avoided Behaviors	*Automatic Thoughts*	*Emotional Reactions*

Comments

Lilly's Self-Image Journal

Date: 7-5-02

Challenging Situation	Response		
	Behavior and Avoided Behaviors	Automatic Thoughts	Emotional Reactions
Getting dressed. Looking in the mirror.	Tried on several outfits; settled on a big, loose dress. My husband was telling me to hurry.	My thighs are so fat and my stomach is fat. I look horrible. I thing they're fatter than they were yesterday.	Disgust, anger with myself, anxiety.
Seeing myself in a bathroom mirror at the movie theater.	I got stuck looking at myself in the mirror. When I came out I asked my husband how I looked. I asked him, "Aren't you embarrassed to be with me?"	I can't stand myself. I won't eat dinner today. I've got to lose more weight. Maybe then I won't look so fat in the stomach. Even in this big dress, I look fat. I look fat in big clothes and in tighter clothes. I can't win.	Disgust, anger with myself
Bathing and getting ready for bed; trying not to look at myself in the mirror.	Bathed and put on my pajamas, trying to avoid the mirror, but I couldn't help sneaking a peak. I weighed myself, even though I dreaded it.	Hurry and get this over with. Maybe I can dress without looking at my disgusting body. I'm hungry, but I won't eat. I need to lose a few pounds, so my stomach and thighs might look decent.	Depressed, over-whelmed, repulsed, hungry

Comments

I look disgusting. My husband says I look fine. In fact, he doesn't want me to lose any more weight. I know he's just saying that, though. He's probably embarrassed to be with me and won't tell me. If I could lose a few more pounds and get my thighs and stomach to look right, everything would be fine. I'd be happy with my body then. Maybe I could try liposuction.

Chart 5b

CHAPTER 6

Deciding to Change

By now, you have a basic understanding of body dysmorphic disorder and body-image dissatisfaction. You've learned about your treatment options, so perhaps you're thinking that self-help is the best option for you, or perhaps you'll be using this book in conjunction with treatment by a mental health professional. You're probably eager (or possibly reluctant) to get started on the process of change. But you have one more step to take before getting into the core of *The BDD Workbook*, the Balanced Image Program. You have to *decide* to change. We will help you examine the information you've collected about your body-image problem and answer these questions:

- Do I want to change?

- Is changing worth the effort?

- Am I ready to change *now*?

The Balanced Image Program is about changing the ways in which you see yourself and think about your body. In recent years researchers have studied how people change, and they have developed a number of important ideas. We will review this new information about change so you can better answer the questions above.

 ## Image Balancing Strategy

Fear, doubt, excuses, and denial are chains that keep you enslaved to your image imbalance. Confronting and refuting your fears will loosen those chains.

Reasons for Not Changing Now

You are probably experiencing many fears and doubts about changing. You may even be tempted to put this book in the back corner of a shelf. But don't do it—not yet anyway. Instead, let's examine some of those fears and doubts.

"My problem's not so bad."

If you truly believed this, you wouldn't be reading this book. Or perhaps you are reading this book only because a relative, friend, or therapist urged you to read it—they see that you have a problem, but you don't. The Balanced Image Program will help you discover the consequences of your views and beliefs about body image. You may decide that you don't need to make any changes, or you may identify some negative consequences and areas that are in need of change. To change or not to change? Examine the facts, then make your decision.

"I've been this way for years. I can't change."

You weren't able to change in the past. You may have tried several times, but you didn't succeed in sticking to your plan. This doesn't mean you can't change now. In the past, you did not have all the tools we describe in this book. In reading this book you will learn the methods and skills you need to initiate changes.

When you say you can't change, you most likely mean that you *don't want to* change. Most people don't like the idea of changing anything. We are comfortable with familiar behaviors; they give us security and a sense of normalcy. However, once change is under way, we learn to accept the new behaviors; eventually they become as comfortable as the old behaviors were.

"Changing is too hard."

Yes, change is difficult. Significant change involves time, effort, and commitment. In most cases it will also mean some discomfort for you and perhaps for those you love. In this chapter you will decide whether the effort is worth the results. Do the advantages of changing outweigh the advantages of staying the same? You don't have to decide now. Consider the facts as you discover them, and then make an informed decision.

"I don't have time to make changes."

We all dedicate our time to the things that are important to us. You've heard the phrase, "Time is money." In a way, it is true—we spend time like we spend money. The payoff, or result, needs to be worth the time spent to achieve it. But as we said earlier, you don't have to decide yet; read on and gather the facts, then determine whether you are willing to dedicate some time to change. Find out if the payoff will be worth your effort and time. In addition, consider the fact that living with body-image problems usually involves quite a bit of time—you'll probably save time by changing.

"This is not the right time to change—maybe later."

There will never be a perfect time to change. You've probably heard the saying, "People only change when they hit rock bottom." But we don't have to wait for a crisis to make changes. In fact, making a change can sometimes prevent a crisis. Don't wait for the perfect circumstances. Life is full of problems and complications. When today's problems straighten out, other problems will provide you with another reason to postpone change.

Even if you do believe the saying about hitting rock bottom, how will you decide where the bottom is? Whenever you decide to change, when you decide that the problem has gone on long enough, that is your bottom. As Alcoholics Anonymous participants know, some people have a higher "bottom" than others do.

"I'm afraid I'll fail."

What if you try to change and you fail? We believe you won't fail, but what if you do? Think of this as a grand experiment, and you have the research of many others, who have conducted similar experiments, to draw on. There is no failure or success in an experiment, only a result. When we don't get the expected result from one experiment, we can go on to life's next experiment. Thomas Edison said, "Results! Why man, I have gotten a lot of results. I know several thousand things that won't work." What's the worst thing that could happen? You might not change much, but you will know you tried.

"I can't change as long as the people around me remain the same."

You can't control the behavior of others, but you can control your own behavior. The culture you live in will remain the same. Those closest to you may not change much. They might not even like your changes. Or they might appreciate the new you. Perhaps others will follow your example. You could be a trendsetter! Even if those around you continue down the same path, you can choose to change your direction. Many people with BDD and related problems are very worried about what others think of their appearance or defect. Working on the program in this book won't change what other people think about your appearance, but it can change how you think about what they think.

Image Balancing Strategy

Don't let fears and doubts hold you back. Decide now to refute your reasons for avoiding change. Keep adding and evaluating reasons over the next few days.

"I don't think I could stand the change."

This book is about making big changes in your self-image, changes that may be painful. Anxiety, depression, grief, and even anger are normal reactions to change. We believe that you can withstand these feelings. And we've built coping strategies into the Balanced Image Program to help you deal with these painful feelings. But what if you can't stand it? What if the anxiety or depression becomes severe and nothing you learn here helps? Even if your worst fears came true, you would still have options. You could return to your old path, or you could get further help, perhaps by joining a support group or by seeking professional help. Acknowledging your fears will help you face them and help you achieve your goals.

Dr. Claiborn sometimes works with people who have chronic pain. At some point during the therapy, many will say, "I can't stand the pain!" Dr. Claiborn is likely to gently ask, "What does it mean, to not be able to stand something?" We all use that expression, or similar ones, in our everyday speech. But what do we really mean? If we say we can't stand something, do we really mean that it is killing us? In fact, we *can* stand it, we stand it all the time, but we don't *like* it.

What Are Your Reasons for Not Changing Now?

What about you? What is holding you back? Perhaps you can relate to one of the reasons listed above. Each of us has our own reasons for not changing now. List your reasons on the following worksheet. Then, for each one, spend some time, as long as needed, to evaluate the reason. Look at evidence that supports or refutes your reasons. We've provided Paul's worksheet as an example.

Stages of Change

We know that people can and do change. We wrote *The BDD Workbook* to help people learn proven techniques to change their body-image-related behaviors and thoughts, either by themselves or with the help of a therapist. James Prochaska, Ph.D., and his colleagues have spent years researching how people change. He's discovered that we change in stages. Dr. Prochaska's model defines these stages and shows that different strategies make sense at different stages (Prochaska, Norcross, and DiClemente 1994). Understanding these stages will help you discover which stage you are in. Having this knowledge will help you determine what to do next as you prepare to change. Follow Paul as he progresses through Prochaska's stages of change.

Precontemplation

People in the *precontemplation stage* do not have an intention to change. Since you are reading this book, you are probably not in this stage (unless you are reading it to help someone else change. In the precontemplation stage people don't see the need to change). Paul's wife was concerned about his anger, but he didn't see it as a problem. Neither of them realized the anger could be related to his body-image concerns.

If you are reading *The BDD Workbook* because you want someone else to change, you need to be aware that the person may still be in the precontemplation stage. The easiest way to determine if others are in this stage is to ask them whether they intend to change in the next six months. If the answer is "no," then they are in the precontemplation stage. Sometimes people will come to a therapist while they are in this stage; however, it is usually because someone else is putting pressure on them to change. They may change the problem behaviors until the pressure is off, but then they usually slip back into their old ways.

Why Not Change Now?

What are your reasons for not changing now?	Evaluate these reasons.

Paul's Why Not Change Now?

What are your reasons for not changing now?	Evaluate these reasons.
I don't have that much of a problem.	My wife is threatening to leave me. At least I can check it out and see if I do have a problem.
I'll finish my anger management class first, and then I'll start the Balanced Image Program.	If I wait, something else could come up, and I'd put it off again. Besides, my anger and my body-image problems are somewhat related.
How will I face my bodybuilding friends?	It's my life. I have to think of my wife and family and the effects of my bodybuilding on them. And on myself! Besides, maybe some of my friends need help too, so my changes might inspire them to change.
It will never work. I will never be able to change.	I really won't know whether I can change or not until I give it a try

Chart 6b

Contemplation

You know you have a problem. You're thinking you really should work on it. You're thinking about changing. This is the *contemplation stage*. Research has shown that people can stay in this stage for years without actually changing (Prochaska, DiClemente, and Norcross 1992). In this stage people are often weighing the pros and cons of the problem and its possible solutions. They are thinking about how much energy it will take to change and the benefits of changing.

After he totaled his car and got into several fights, Paul realized he had a problem. He was also tiring of the bodybuilding and had increasing worries about his body image. He thought about changing occasionally, but he didn't pursue it.

Preparation

In the *preparation stage* people are ready to change and may have made some early efforts to change. Dr. Claiborn likes to tell the following joke to his patients: "How many psychologists does it take to change a lightbulb? Only one, but the bulb has to be ready to change." If you've read this far, perhaps you are in this stage. You purchased *The BDD Workbook* with the intention of changing body-image-related behaviors. You've filled out worksheets and answered questions about your body-image problem. You are collecting information and getting ready to change.

When Paul's wife threatened to leave, he went with her to a marriage counselor. That's when he learned that his anger problem was likely related to the anabolic steroids he had been taking. He began researching the adverse effects of steroid use. Realizing that he had a problem with body image, he also researched BDD and muscle dysmorphia.

Action

The *action stage* is the stage that commonly comes to mind when most people think about changing. In this stage, people are doing things others will recognize as efforts to change. When you are in the action stage you are likely to describe yourself as working hard on the problem and may say things like, "Anyone can talk about changing, but I'm really working on it." A person's work at this stage of change is recognized and often supported or praised by others. Sometimes this recognition is a problem because the work in the earlier and later stages, when you also need support, is ignored.

Paul enlisted his wife's help and worked with his therapist to challenge some of his beliefs about his body image. He decided he needed to change and used cognitive behavioral therapy principles to handle his problems with muscle dysmorphia and BDD.

Maintenance

Many people will not recognize the *maintenance stage* as an active one, but this final stage is very important in preventing relapse. Most people will stay in the maintenance stage for the rest of their lives. In this stage, people need to make changes in long-term patterns in order to stabilize themselves and prevent a return to problem behaviors.

Even when he had reached the maintenance stage, Paul still felt that his muscles weren't as big as he'd like. He continued to review the cognitive behavioral therapy principles he'd learned, in order to remind himself of where he had been and why he had decided to change. He was able to manage his discomfort with his body image using the principles he had learned in therapy. He knew how to recognize risky situations and distorted thinking, so he was able to get himself back on track when necessary.

We know that people don't move through these stages in a straight line. Dr. Prochaska describes the process of change as more of a spiral. Almost everyone has made a New Year's resolution to change a habit, lose weight, or complete some kind of self-improvement project, and almost everyone has slipped back at some point. The embarrassment and shame of failure may lead to our moving all the way back from the action stage to the precontemplation stage. Mark Twain said, "To cease smoking is the easiest thing I ever did. I ought to know because I've done it a thousand times." He was probably cycling back and forth through the contemplation, preparation, and action stages.

Image Balancing Strategy

Make moving into the action stage a short-term goal as you work toward changing your body-image-related behaviors and thoughts.

Change Is a Process

Dr. Prochaska and other researchers have described ten processes of change. Studies have found these processes to be to be important in any effort to change (Prochaska, Norcross, and DiClemente 1995). It is interesting to see how these *processes* of change fit within the *stages* of change.

- **Consciousness raising** involves gaining information about yourself and the behaviors you are trying to change. Reading this book and doing exercises that help you describe your body image are examples of ways to raise your consciousness. This process is important in the precontemplation and contemplation stages of change. If you are reading this because you want to help someone else who seems to be in one of these two stages, then giving that person information, confronting him or her about the effects of the self-image problem, and pointing out when body-image-related behaviors occur may be effective forms of consciousness raising.

- **Emotional arousal** is another important process in the precontemplation and contemplation stages. This involves experiencing and expressing feelings about the problem and its possible solutions. Doing this may help you move from the precontemplation to the contemplation and preparation stages. People with body-image problems are often in a state of distress. This distress can provide motivation to change. It already provides the motivation to do things like check your appearance or find ways to change your appearance. We want you to take that same motivation and channel it toward making a change in how you see yourself.

- **Self-reevaluation** involves assessing how you feel about yourself with respect to your body image. This may include examining your values, identifying what you want to achieve, and deciding how you would like things to be in the future. This process takes place in the contemplation and preparation stages. Some of the questions in this book, especially the ones that ask you to examine your body image and your ideas about its importance to your overall self-image, are designed to help you with self-reevaluation.

- **Environmental reevaluation** is the process of evaluating how your problem affects your physical environment. Considering how it affects other people, your relationships, and your financial well-being are parts of this process. Like self-reevaluation, this happens in the contemplation and preparation stages. Many people with BDD and associated problems will find that their body-image concerns have significant effects on how they relate to others, how they spend their money, and generally how they interact with the world.

- **A commitment** is a choice to act and believe in the ability to change. This process of making a commitment often takes place in the preparation and action stages. You will need to make a commitment to change the way you think and act if you are going to modify how your body-image problem affects your life.

- **A helping relationship** can be an important part of making a change. Therapists are trained to pay attention to these relationships, and many types of therapy utilize the helping relationship as a major ingredient in change. If you are trying to change without the help of a therapist, being open with someone you trust and discussing your body-image problem and related behaviors that you are trying to change can be helpful. Self-help groups can provide this kind of relationship. The helping relationship seems to be most important in the action and maintenance stages.

- **Counterconditioning** is a change process that is likely to be recommended by a behavior therapist, but often people discover it on their own. This involves substituting alternatives for the problem behavior. Using relaxation, meditation, and positive self-statements are examples. This change process is most important in the action and maintenance stages. *The BDD Workbook* includes several counterconditioning exercises.

- **Environment control** involves avoiding or changing the stimuli that elicit the problem behavior. Like counterconditioning, this process is used in the action and maintenance stages. Environmental control could involve removing mirrors or bathroom scales from your home or canceling subscriptions to certain magazines.

- **Reward,** also called reinforcement, is a very powerful tool. You might reward yourself or be rewarded by others for making changes. Reinforcements, or rewards, are effective whether they come from yourself or from others. This is important to keep in mind if you are trying to get somebody else to change. Reinforcement management is important in the action and maintenance stages.

- **Social liberation** involves efforts to promote alternatives to particular behaviors or viewpoints in society at large. This can include actions such as advocating for the rights of others, helping other people battle body-image problems, and speaking out about some of the destructive messages regarding body-image and beauty in our culture.

What Stage Are You In?

Now that we have explained some of the principles of change, it is time for you to pick up your pencil again. Let's look at where you are in the stages of change.

What stage of change are you in right now? _____

_____

Now, review the change processes described above and list the ones that could best help you, given your current stage. _____

_____

_____

Are You Ready to Change?

Why change *now*? It may seem like a silly question, but something must be motivating you if you have gotten this far. Stating your reasons to change can help solidify the motivation to change. Sometimes a particular incident or an upcoming event makes people want to change. For Paul, it was his wife's threat to leave him and his discovery that his anger problem could be the result of the anabolic steroids he had taken. We've included Paul's reasons for changing as an example.

List some reasons for changing now. Include reasons that might not have been true before. _____

_____

_____

_____

_____

_____

_____

_____

Paul:

List some reasons for changing now. Include reasons that might not have been true before. _My wife is threatening to leave me because of my angry outbursts and because I've hit her. My neighbor and my brother are mad at me and worried about the change in my personality. My car insurance has been increased three times. I'm not making as much money working at the gym as I did working at the bank. I'm always thinking about my body's appearance and comparing myself with other bodybuilders. My children are learning the wrong things about appearance from me. I'm afraid they will grow up thinking body appearance is more important than other aspects of self-image._

Here's another question that may seem strange: What are the advantages or benefits of *not* changing? We'll put it another way: What do you get out of your preoccupation with body image? Fill in the boxes in the Change Advantages and Disadvantages worksheet. Then look at your results. Are the advantages of changing more important to you than the disadvantages of changing? If so, you are ready to make some changes. If not, you may not yet be ready to change. Continue reading *The BDD Workbook*, keeping your Self-Image Journal, and adding to your Change Advantages and Disadvantages worksheet. We've provided Paul's worksheet as an example.

 Image Balancing Strategy

Why do you want to change *now*? When your motivation is at its lowest, review your answers and remind yourself of *why* you want to change.

Now, take a look at your disadvantages of changing. Most of your worries about changing will likely be dealt with as you go through the Balanced Image Program. Paul did lose some of his muscle mass because his body took on a more normal shape, unaltered by anabolic steroids. He was surprised to find that his wife was more pleased with his new body shape. Paul didn't stop working out altogether; he learned to exercise for physical fitness rather than appearance. He discovered that his health improved when he exercise moderately rather than to excess. Some of his friends at the gym became more distant when he worked out less, but two of his friends decided that they were putting too much emphasis on body image and decided to change too. In addition, he rebuilt relationships with other friends.

Ready?

Remember the three questions we asked at the beginning of this chapter? We've answered the first two questions, "Do I want to change?" and "Is changing worth the effort?" The last question might be the hardest: "Am I ready to change *now*?" If your answer is "yes," you are in the preparation or action stage, and you are ready to begin the Balanced Image Program, presented in chapters 7 through 15. Now is the time to make a commitment.

Pick a date on which you will start reading and applying the tools in the Balanced Image Program. Write the date here. _____

Remember that helping relationships are important. Make a list of people who can give you support as you change your behaviors. _____

Tell your support people about your commitment and let them know how they can help. Explain how they can reinforce change. What are some specific things they can do to reinforce your efforts? _____

Recognizing that you have a problem with body image and making a decision to change are important preliminary steps. Continue to keep your Self-Image Journal as you read chapter 7, the beginning of the Balanced Image Program. You will learn some very important skills that will help you throughout the process of change—you will learn how to relax.

 Image Balancing Strategy

Make a copy of your Change Advantages and Disadvantages worksheet and keep it in a conspicuous place. Review it when change seems almost impossible.

Change Advantages and Disadvantages

Advantages of Changing	Disadvantages of Changing

Paul's Change Advantages and Disadvantages

Advantages of Changing	Disadvantages of Changing
I wouldn't have so much anxiety about my appearance.	I'd lose some of the muscle mass I gained by taking steroids.
I could concentrate on more important matters, instead of thinking so much about my appearance.	I might lose interest in my appearance so much that I might stop working out and get fat.
I'd probably spend less time working out.	My friends at the gym would lose their respect for me and we probably wouldn't be such good friends.
I'd have more time to spend with my family and doing other things I enjoy.	
My wife and I would have a better relationship, and she'd be less worried about me.	
I could rebuild relationships with old friends, my brother, and my neighbor.	
I might be more satisfied with my appearance.	
My children would learn from my example, they'd see the dangers of putting too much focus on appearance, and they would see the importance of other parts of self-image.	
I'd spend less money on supplements.	
I'd be less tempted to injure my health with steroids.	

Chart 6c

Part II

The Balanced Image Program

CHAPTER 7

Relaxation

You will use relaxation training in your Balanced Image Program. Learning to relax can be useful in handling many situations and behavior problems. Relaxation training is an important aspect of habit reversal, a technique developed by behavior therapists that is very useful for working on problems like skin picking. (We'll discuss habit reversal in chapter 11.) Most people with body-image problems experience anxiety in social situations or even at home when they are thinking about their bodies. Relaxation training is a tool you can use to help manage any anxiety, no matter what its cause.

Alfred's anxiety about the appearance of his arms was sometimes quite severe. Going out in public had become so distressing that he had begun to stay home more and more. Relaxation helped him handle the stress of going out. After a few weeks of practicing daily relaxation he was able to make use of what is known as *cue-controlled relaxation*. He could achieve a state of greater relaxation even when he was in public. Alfred learned that his efforts to hold his arms in just the right position so they would look right were actually sources of considerable tension. His muscles had often ached and felt tense from such posing. When he recognized this he found that he was able to relax his shoulders and arms more readily.

Relaxation will also play a role in changing body-image-related behaviors. You've probably developed some unhealthy or negative ways of coping with anxiety about your body image. Since you will be taking these coping methods away you will need to develop other ways of dealing with stress and anxiety. We will teach you some relaxation exercises, and eventually you will be able to use one or more of them whenever you feel the urge to engage in your old coping methods. First, though, you will need to practice relaxation for several minutes a day. The more you practice, the more you will be prepared to relax when the urge to engage in the problem behavior hits.

Morgan's BDD-related behaviors took up hours every day. She shopped for creams to hide the dark circles under her eyes and the scar on her chin, applied the creams, checked the results over and over, studied her image in the mirror, and pored over beauty magazines searching for new solutions. Part of Morgan's Balanced Image Program involved replacing these behaviors with other activities. Relaxation exercises helped her cope with the anxiety she experienced and gave her a pleasant activity with which to replace some of the problem behaviors that had become habits.

 Image Balancing Strategy

Relaxation can bring relief from anxiety, stress, nervousness, and worry and help you focus on the Balanced Image Program.

Relaxation Methods

You've heard the old doctor's order, "Take two aspirin and call me in the morning." Well, relaxation training is sometimes called "the aspirin of behavioral treatments." Relaxation is considered to be good for nearly everyone.

You may think you already know how to relax. You watch TV, read, sleep, take long walks, eat "comfort foods," or drink alcohol. While these activities may be relaxing in their own way, we are referring to a different kind of relaxation. Our goal is to relax our bodies and minds. Relaxation exercises can help you have more energy, control anxiety, and even lower blood pressure. Below we have provided three relaxation methods. Choose the one that most appeals to you or try them all.

IMPORTANT NOTE: If you are taking medications for anxiety, diabetes, or high blood pressure, consult your doctor before beginning relaxation training. He or she may want to adjust your medication dosage as you reduce your stress, anxiety, and tension. If you have a physical problem such as osteoporosis, heart or lung disease, or other disorder, there is a slight chance one or more of these exercises could have adverse affects on your condition. Ask your doctor to tell you which relaxation exercise would be best for you. Occasionally people with anxiety problems become panicky when trying to relax. If this occurs you will want to discuss this with a mental health professional.

Abdominal Breathing

How do you breathe? Take notice of your breathing style next time you are nervous. Does your chest rise and fall, or does your abdomen do most of the moving? Are your shoulders tense and inching upward with every breath? Do your muscles feel tight? Abdominal breathing can help. Cherry has vocal-cord tightness, which sometimes gives her a hoarse voice and makes her stutter, especially when she is nervous. When speaking in public, she had a habit of tensing her shoulders and breathing with her chest, rather than with her abdominal muscles. A friend who was a member of Toastmasters advised her to relax her shoulders and slow her breathing. She did this and practiced abdominal breathing. As a result, her speaking voice improved and she felt less nervous when she spoke.

When your shoulders and abdominal muscles are tight, you tend not to use your abdomen to breathe. Because you are not filling your lungs fully, you probably don't get enough air. To compensate, you breathe faster, with shallow breaths. The nervous, anxious feelings worsen. After practicing abdominal breathing, you will learn to recognize your nervous breathing and switch to a more relaxed breathing style. Practice the following exercise for five to ten minutes daily.

1. Lie in a comfortable position. Breathe normally for five breaths. Does your chest move up and down with each breath, or does your abdomen move? If you can't tell, rest one hand on your chest and one on your abdomen. Which one moves most? If you still can't tell, try resting a book on your abdomen. Does it move up and down? If your abdomen moves up and down and your chest stays fairly still, you're doing great. If you find your chest is moving more than your abdomen, try to make your abdomen do more of the work. Intentionally push your stomach out as you breathe in and let it fall back into place as you breathe out. This may feel strange at first, but with some practice it should become more comfortable.

2. Close your eyes and breathe in, using your abdomen. Breathe in deeply, pushing your stomach up, keeping your chest relatively still.

3. Take several slow, deep breaths, then open your eyes and look at or place your hand on your abdomen. Is your abdomen rising and falling? Continue slow, deep breathing.

4. If you're still mostly using your chest, try pressing down gently on your abdomen as you exhale. Still having trouble? Lie down on the floor face down with your arms at your sides. Push your stomach into the floor as you breathe in. Remember, it takes time to change nervous breathing to relaxed breathing.

5. When you have learned to use abdominal breathing while lying down, practice abdominal breathing sitting, then standing.

6. Once you have learned to breathe this way, try doing it whenever you find yourself in a stressful situation. Recognize your nervous breathing and switch to the relaxed abdominal breathing pattern you have learned.

7. Take time to practice this way of breathing during the course of the day; when you are stopped at a traffic light or standing in line at the supermarket, take a few of these breaths.

Progressive Muscle Relaxation

The body often responds to anxiety and stress by tensing the muscles. Progressive muscle relaxation is an effective way of bringing about a state of relaxation and becoming aware of this muscle tension. It involves tightening your muscles beyond normal tension, then relaxing them. This process helps you to focus attention on what the muscles are doing and leads to a general state of relaxation. In this exercise, you will learn to tighten and relax your muscles, one group of muscles at a time. For best results, devote at least fifteen minutes a day to the practice of progressive muscle relaxation.

1. Sit in a comfortable, supportive chair with your feet on the floor, or lie comfortably with your arms at your sides and your legs stretched out straight.

2. Take three slow, deep breaths. (Review the above instructions on abdominal breathing for the best way to breathe during relaxation.)

3. Tighten the muscles in your hands and forearms. Make a tight fist and hold it for ten seconds. Focus your attention on the way the muscles in your arms and hands feel. Relax your hands and arms for fifteen seconds. Focus on how different it feels as the muscles relax. Notice the sensations in your hands and arms.

4. Tighten your forearms by flexing your wrists and your upper arms in the same way—tighten for ten seconds, relax for fifteen seconds. Focus on the sensations in the muscles when they are tense and relaxed.

5. Tighten the muscles of your forehead and squeeze your eyes shut. Hold this tension for ten seconds and focus on what you feel in your face. Now let those same muscles relax and for the next fifteen seconds pay attention to the change in feelings in your forehead and around your eyes.

6. Tighten the muscles of your jaw and neck and focus on the feelings associated with the tension in these muscles. Hold the tension for ten seconds. Now release the tension, letting your jaw relax. You may want to open your mouth a little. Notice the change in sensation in your jaw and neck, focusing on it for the next fifteen seconds.

7. Pull your shoulders up toward your head and tense the muscles there for ten seconds. At the same time tighten the muscles of the chest. You may want to hold your breath. Let your shoulders drop, breathe easily and slowly, and let all of the tension go from your chest. Spend fifteen seconds focusing on how different your shoulders and chest feel when they are relaxed.

8. Tighten your stomach. Imagine someone is about to punch you—try to make your belly hard. Hold that tension for ten seconds and focus on the feeling in your abdomen. Let the muscles relax, and breathe from the diaphragm, letting your stomach move in a relaxed fashion as you breathe. Focus on the difference in the sensations for fifteen seconds.

9. Tighten the muscles of your lower back and buttocks. Hold that tension for ten seconds and focus on how the muscles feel. Now let yourself relax and sink down into your chair. Feel the change in sensation as the muscles relax. Focus on these sensations for fifteen seconds.

10. Tighten the muscles of your thighs. Hold this tension for ten seconds and focus on how your upper legs feel. Now let them relax and notice the change in sensation for fifteen seconds. Do you experience discomfort with the tension? Is there warmth associated with the relaxation?

11. Tighten the muscles of your lower leg and flex your feet so that you move your toes toward your shinbone. Hold this tension for ten seconds and focus on the sensations in your lower legs. Now let your feet drop back into place and let your lower legs relax. Notice the change in sensation as your legs and feet relax. Focus on it for fifteen seconds.

12. Are you relaxed? Scan your body, one muscle group at a time. If you feel tension anywhere, repeat the tense-and-relax cycle for that muscle group.

When you've practiced progressive relaxation daily for a week or so and feel comfortable with it, go through the tensing and relaxing of each muscle group a bit more quickly. Note that the recommended ten and fifteen seconds are guidelines. You don't need to time yourself precisely. You may choose to modify the exercise to fit your particular preferences. For example, you may find it helpful to tighten and relax one extremity at a time, or to modify the muscle groups so that they make sense to you. Try practicing progressive muscle relaxation while standing. Now you have a relaxation method you can use any time you experience tension and stress.

Many people find it easiest to learn this method if they record the instructions and play the recording during the exercise. The tone of voice and speaking pace should be relaxed and calm. If you don't like the sound of your voice, have someone else record the instructions. On the tape, tell yourself to tense and relax individual muscles in the order given above. When you have been practicing progressive relaxation for a few weeks, you can try another variation. Simply omit the tension of the muscle groups and go down your body thinking about each of the muscle groups and letting the muscles relax. Think about the muscles feeling heavy, warm, and relaxed.

You can move on to cue-controlled relaxation next. First, do the progressive muscle relaxation exercise. After scanning your body for any remaining tension begin to repeat the word "relax" with each breath. Practice this for a few minutes after each session of progressive muscle relaxation. After you have done this for a week or more try repeating the word "relax" with your breathing when you find yourself in a tense situation. With practice, using this technique should allow you to bring on a state of greater relaxation on cue.

Meditation

People have been practicing meditation for at least five thousand years. Most religions teach some type of meditation as a spiritual discipline. Prayer, chanting, the study of Scripture, and worship can all be forms of meitation. While pursuing the meditative practices of your religious tradition can bring about spiritual and physical refreshment, this is not the type of meditation described here. In addition to producing relaxation, reducing stress, and relieving anxiety, meditation can also influence your metabolic rate, decrease your heart rate, increase your alertness, decrease desire to use alcohol and drugs, and reduce chronic anxiety. Meditation has been shown to be helpful for a number of problems, including headaches, chronic pain, and high blood pressure (Benson and Stuart 1993).

Still, you may have concerns that meditation is in conflict with your religious beliefs. If you are uncomfortable with it, consider trying one of the other relaxation techniques or a meditation tec hnique taught within your religion. For a comprehensive description of Christian meditation, relaxation, stress reduction, and anxiety relief, Cherry recommends *The Anxiety Cure* by Archibald D. Hart. He also has a relaxation tape available. You can find more information about these and other resources in the last section of this book. You can also discuss this with your clergyman or other trusted advisor, showing him or her the discussion here.

Meditation for psychological and emotional benefits can be divided into two types: concentrative meditation and external awareness meditation. Mindfulness is an example of external awareness meditation. Below, Dr. Claiborn offers an example of concentrative meditation. The goal is to restrict awareness of the outside world by focusing on a word, mental image, or phrase.

1. Do what you can to reduce noise or other distractions around you. If that's not possible, you may want to play soft music or nature sounds. Sit in a comfortable chair and close your eyes.

2. If you're feeling tense or nervous, spend a few minutes doing progressive muscle relaxation or abdominal breathing.

3. Focus your attention on a word or a mental image. Try to make it the focus of your attention, but without turning it into a struggle.

4. When other thoughts come to mind, let them float on by. Don't try to push them out of your mind, but don't focus on them either; just accept the thoughts (or perhaps thank your mind for sharing them) and then let them go. If a thought or worry just won't leave your mind, stop and write it down; now you can let go of it.

5. Focus on a word or phrase. It can be a neutral word, or a phrase that has special meaning for you, like "praise God," "relax," or "be still." Dr. Claiborn often recommends the word "calm." Cherry's preference is a Bible verse.

6. Aloud or in your mind, say the chosen focus word or phrase with every breath you let out. You may want to stretch the word out for the entire length of the exhaled breath.

7. When thoughts pop into your head, gently remind yourself to stay focused on your word and your mental image. Let the thought float on by.

8. Practice this type of meditation for ten to fifteen minutes daily. If it seems very hard at first, start with just five minutes. When you feel nervous or stressed, do a shortened version of this exercise. With time, you'll be able to bring on a relaxed state in just a few minutes.

Mindfulness

We discussed Ellen Langer's study of mindfulness and mindlessness in chapter 2. In the context used here, *mindfulness* is a form of external awareness meditation. The purpose of this type of meditation is the opposite of the purpose of concentrative meditation techniques. Instead of restricting awareness of the outside world, the object is to increase your awareness of the outside world. In *The Anxiety Cure*, Archibald. Hart (1999) writes, "the Benedictine monks have a discipline of 'listening' to the world. They believe God speaks through nature and history, that God is manifest in *all* of His creation. For example, when you peel and eat an orange, you pay attention to all its attributes: its fragrance, its texture, its taste . . . Similarly, the Quakers have a practice of 'listening with the heart.' Silence is used extensively to aid in 'hearing' what God has to say to your heart." He points out that "the stress-lowering value of the meditation doesn't necessarily come from the content of the meditation, but from the process of meditation. It slows you down, for one thing. In addition, it helps you to control your thoughts."

Much of the writing about mindfulness is associated with Zen Buddhism. While some people use mindfulness as a spiritual practice, the use here is therapeutic and focuses on the physical effects of relaxing the body, reducing stress, relieving anxiety, and learning self-acceptance. Mindfulness is a powerful tool that you can apply to your efforts to change. In Zen Buddhist teachings, stories are often used to make a point or help convey concepts. The story below is one that Dr. Claiborn often uses to explain the concept of mindfulness.

Once upon a time there was a monk on a journey through the mountains. He was walking along when a tiger appeared and prepared to attack him. The monk ran for his life. He came to a cliff, which he tried to climb down to escape the tiger. He had not climbed very far before it became very clear that he could climb no further without plunging to his death on the rocks below. He could climb back up and be killed by the tiger or drop to the rocks below and die. As he clung to the rocks considering his fate, he noticed a strawberry plant growing out of the cliff. There was one small ripe strawberry on the plant. The monk picked and ate the strawberry. He thought, "How delicious."

When Dr. Claiborn tells this story to his patients he sometimes has to say, "That is the end of the story." This story, with its somewhat unexpected ending, reminds us to be mindful. We are accustomed to paying attention to urgent problems and events as we go through our lives, which can cause us to miss some of the more ordinary but wonderful aspects of life. The monk, faced with horrible choices, stops long enough to enjoy the strawberry in a mindful way. He focuses his attention on the experience of eating the strawberry without preoccupation with his past or future. He doesn't complain about the unfairness of being chased by the tiger or the deadly sharpness of the rocks below. He doesn't bemoan the meager strawberry harvest. He stops and experiences the present moment in all its reality and does not make judgments. This is the essence of mindfulness.

Sometimes people have difficulty understanding this story or seeing how it is relevant to problems like body image. Think of it this way: The tiger can be thought of as any stress or threat in our lives. There are times when problem solving or other efforts do not work. These are times when we need to accept things as they are. Acceptance is a difficult concept for many of us. Through mindfulness we can get to the point of truly accepting our problems by becoming part of the present experience rather than trying to live in the past or the future.

In his book, *Brain Lock*, Dr. Jeffrey Schwartz (1996) describes the use of mindfulness as a central technique for dealing with obsessions. The concept of mindfulness is further described and used in chapters 9, 11, and 12. For now, we'll try a couple of exercises to help you learn how to be more mindful.

Breathing Mindfully

Sit in a comfortable position for about five minutes with your mind focused on your breathing. Notice how you breathe. Are you breathing through your mouth or nose or both? If you are breathing through your nose, are you breathing through one nostril more than the other? Notice the sensations that accompany your breathing. Simply observe how it feels to breathe. Do not judge how you are, breathing but become an impartial scientist observing and noticing. When you pay attention to your breathing, it may change. If this happens, observe it but don't try to prevent it.

While you are focusing on your breathing other thoughts will come into your mind. This doesn't mean you aren't doing the exercise right—it happens to everyone. Don't try to push the thoughts away; simply observe them and let them go. Return to observing your breathing. Practice this every day for a week before trying the next mindfulness exercise.

More Mindfulness

If you think about the monk and the strawberry it may be clear to you that almost any experience can be turned into an exercise in mindfulness. When you have gained some comfort with the mindful breathing exercise, try to use the same impartial observance with other everyday experiences. Start with activities you do every day. Eating a meal mindfully can be a great new experience. You can notice the textures, flavors, and colors of a meal, no matter how ordinary it is. Try walking mindfully, noticing how walking feels. What are your feet, legs, and arms doing? How do you shift your weight? What do you need to do to maintain your balance and keep going where you want to go? There are thousands of experiences you can try to experience mindfully. Remember not to judge, but simply to observe. Include in the observation how you are feeling, without judging yourself on how you think you are supposed to feel.

One of the hardest things to do when practicing being mindful is to avoid getting caught up in the thoughts that come into your mind. These thoughts can include judgments, worries about how mindful you are being, and thoughts about problems that you are having in your life. Simply thank your mind for sharing—this is a nonjudgmental approach. Think of your mind as a tree full of monkeys. The monkeys chatter incessantly, jump around from branch to branch, and even throw things at passersby. The monkeys are trying to get your attention, to draw your focus away, but all that noise and excitement is not really important. Everyone becomes distracted by internal thoughts at times, but we need to remember that these thoughts are like a bunch of noisy monkeys and they don't have any important messages for us at that moment.

Dr. Marsha Linehan has developed a treatment for people who seem to hate themselves, such as those with borderline personality disorder. One of the core elements of this treatment is mindfulness training. Dr. Linehan offers a set of guidelines for mindfulness that we will paraphrase below (Linehan 1993).

1. Observe your experiences. Just notice what is happening. Have a "Teflon" mind; don't let thoughts stick. Just watch your thoughts float by like clouds in the sky.

2. Describe your experience to yourself. You might say things like, "I am filled with sadness," or "My stomach feels tight."

3. Enter into experiences and become fully involved in the present.

4. Suspend judgment. Don't evaluate or criticize your experience or thoughts. They are not good or bad; they simply are. Try to accept each moment, thought, or sensation.

5. Do one thing at a time and do it mindfully. Eat when you are eating and walk when you are walking. Even worry can be done mindfully.

6. Focus on accepting what is, not what is fair or unfair, should or should not be.

Dr. Claiborn has listed books about mindfulness in the Resources section of this book. He recommends *Wherever You Go, There You Are: Mindfulness Meditation in Everyday Life*, by Jon Kabat-Zinn.

 Image Balancing Strategy

Choose a relaxation technique and practice it daily while you are working on the Balanced Image Program.

Practicing daily relaxation exercises will help relieve your anxiety, stress, tension, and boredom. As a result, you will help reduce the urges to engage in behaviors that perpetuate your negative body image. Choose a relaxation technique and begin practicing it daily. If that one doesn't work well for you, choose another one. Being relaxed will also help you work through the next two chapters. We'll help you examine your thoughts concerning body image and replace them with more realistic thoughts.

CHAPTER 8

Changing Automatic Thoughts That Affect Body Image

H umans are thinking creatures. We are continuously thinking and processing information. Think about an activity that you do every day. Mentally review each step of the activity. What do you do first? What do you do next? What thoughts are involved in the activity? Let's consider what Alfred did each morning when he got up. He would spend quite a bit of time looking at his arms in the mirror. He'd pose with his arms in different positions, trying to decide if he could even try going out that morning and what he could do to make himself look less repulsive. This process went on each day in very much the same way. He didn't realize that there was a lot of thinking involved, so he never stopped to look at those thoughts carefully.

Alfred's Body-Image-Related Behaviors, Thoughts, and Emotions worksheet illustrates the behaviors, thoughts, and emotional reactions he experienced when he got up in the morning. As you look at his automatic thoughts you will see how much they contributed to Alfred's anxiety about his appearance.

Most of our behaviors and thoughts are based on what we've learned in the past. When you drive your car, you must recall how to drive, the meaning of traffic lights and signs, and how to get where you are going. When you bake a cake, you must remember where the ingredients and utensils are, how to read a recipe, how to turn on the oven, and what the timer's buzzer means. Each of these activities involves the recall of previous learning.

We perform these activities automatically, without much awareness. In addition, we can drive a car or bake a cake while listening to the radio, conversing with others, answering the phone, or thinking about other activities. We all process a massive amount of information through automatic thinking. Just imagine driving a car, baking a cake, or operating a computer *without* automatically remembering your past learning! If we had to pay attention to every detail of our everyday activities, we would get very little done. It would be impossible to perform our daily activities without using some type of automatic processing.

Alfred's Body-Image-Related Behaviors, Thoughts, and Emotions

Activity or situation: Get out of bed and look in mirror.

Step	Behavior	Automatic Thought	Emotional Reaction
1	Wake up, sit up in bed.	Another day with my disgusting body.	Depressed, tired, even though I just woke up.
2	Weigh myself.	I've lost a pound since last week. I look scrawny. I need to eat more. Maybe a new supplement would help.	Disappointed.
3	Look in mirror, pose with my arms at my side, then folded across my chest, waving.	I'm disgusting. I can't go out today, not looking like this. I would be too embarrassed. Even my wrists are puny and ugly.	Disgust, anxiety.
4	Try on a shirt, then another shirt.	I can't completely cover these repulsive arms. Maybe I could wait until late tonight, then go to the store. No, I'll ask Mom to pick things up for me.	Depressed, resigned, disgust, anxiety.
5	Try on a jacket, then a bulky sweater.	Maybe this will work, if the sweater is loose enough, no one will notice my arms. No, even then, they look too small. And look at my wrists. They still show, even with the jacket on.	Anxiety, disgust, revulsion.

Chart 8a

Alfred's Previously Learned Behaviors and Thoughts worksheet show his automatic thoughts and behaviors that involved things he had learned previously. These include his own thoughts about himself, including his appearance. It is clear that the kinds of things Alfred thought contributed to how he ended up feeling.

Alfred's Previously Learned Behaviors and Thoughts

What automatic thoughts did you have that were based on previous learning? _____
I remembered what I weighed last week and that I was unhappy with that weight.
I remembered that having small arms makes me feel puny, that I've tried to eat more and still lost a pound. I remembered that I usually weigh myself and look at my arms in the mirror first thing in the morning.

Chart 8b

We can understand the link between thoughts and feelings by using a simple model. This diagram shows that it is not events that lead to emotional reactions, but what we think about them. This means that our automatic thoughts lead to our emotional responses.

Events   →   Automatic thoughts   →   Emotional reaction

Core beliefs

When Alfred looked in the mirror and saw his arms (the event) he would automatically think, "I have a disgustingly ugly arms. If I go out looking like this everyone will stare and see what a monster I am." The emotional reactions to these thoughts were fear and disgust, or shame.

You can think of beliefs as kind of a template that shapes automatic thoughts. Alfred may have had a few core beliefs that were active here, such as "My self-worth depends on what I look like" and "I am ugly." As you can see, it would be important for him to change both the automatic thoughts and the core beliefs in order to help himself feel better. Is the same true for you? It depends. If you have a mild body-image problem you may well have some core beliefs that are actually helpful, and you will need to use them, instead of your unhelpful core beliefs, to mold your automatic thoughts. If you have a more serious body-image problem, such as BDD, you may have to work hard to change your core beliefs or develop new ones.

Now try to complete your own Body-Image-Related Behaviors, Thoughts, and Emotions worksheet and Previously Learned Behaviors and Thoughts worksheet. If it seems too difficult to complete these worksheets using a body-image-related activity, first use any activity that you do almost daily, then tackle a body-image-related activity. Make seven copies of the blank worksheets and complete at least one set every day for a week. We will be asking how to do a similar exercise in the next chapter.

Body-Image-Related Behaviors, Thoughts, and Emotions

Activity or situation:

Step	Behavior	Automatic Thought	Emotional Reaction

Chart 8c

The Body-Image-Related Behaviors, Thoughts, and Emotions worksheet is similar to the Self-Image Journal you have been keeping. The important difference is that you are breaking down an activity or situation into its steps and examining the behaviors, thoughts, and emotions involved at each step. As you continue keeping your Self-Image Journal consider how activities and situations are made up of many steps or stages. Often, thoughts and emotions escalate along the way.

Previously Learned Behaviors and Thoughts

What automatic thoughts did you have that were based on previous learning?

_____

_____

_____

_____

_____

Chart 8d

Cognitive Behavioral Therapy For Body-Image Problems

Cognitive behavioral therapy is used to help people change the way they think and act so they can change the way they feel. Many important techniques used in cognitive behavioral therapy focus on the type of automatic processing we described above. Cognitive behavioral therapy based on methods developed by Dr. Aaron Beck and others has been used effectively to treat a broad range of problems, including depression and anxiety. In fact, in many cases it works as well as—or even better than—medication! Cognitive behavioral therapy is also effective in preventing relapse, or the return of symptoms, for years after treatment.

Consider Duncan's problems with skin picking. This behavior usually began when he looked in a mirror and saw a blemish. His automatic thoughts would include the following: "There's a spot . . . it has a ragged edge and looks ugly . . . I need to smooth it . . . if I have a blemish I am imperfect and repulsive." This led to an emotional response of distress since he was thinking of himself as imperfect and repulsive. Thinking of one's self as repulsive would upset anyone. In fact, Duncan had many automatic thoughts about the meaning of looking the way that he thought he did. Before he was able to examine these thoughts, Duncan's hand would be on his face. Other automatic thoughts would go through his mind, such as "I know I shouldn't pick. I don't need to do this."

Then he'd give into the urge and think, "I have to fix it. I'll just pick this one spot . . . smoothing this spot will make it look better." These last few thoughts are what we call *permission-giving thoughts*. Duncan didn't completely believe them and had other, conflicting thoughts, like "I am weak and can't control myself," which contributed to his feeling guilty and angry.

Be especially alert to *permission-giving thoughts*. They make us much more likely to follow through with the action we are contemplating. Automatic thoughts whiz through our minds in a shorthand form. Most people aren't aware of many of their thoughts and may claim that they don't think *anything*, they just act. However, we know this isn't how our brains work. We think, then we act. In upsetting situations, the thoughts are there and gone before we have had a chance to consciously process them. Therein lies the problem.

If your thinking is so automatic, how can you change the pattern of your thoughts? Using cognitive therapy skills, you can slow these thoughts by paying more attention to them. As you look at them, you can make important changes in your automatic thoughts, then change the way you act in response to the thoughts. Changing your thoughts and actions will also bring about changes in your emotions. Completing the Body-Image-Related Behaviors, Thoughts, and Feelings worksheet is the beginning of this process.

Fill out a Body-Image-Related Behaviors, Thoughts, and Feelings worksheet and a Previously Learned Behaviors and Thoughts worksheet whenever you find yourself upset about your appearance, at least once a day for the next week. Describe the situation or activity and list the steps, then record your automatic thoughts and emotional reactions. You will probably find that it becomes progressively easier to identify your automatic thoughts and emotional reactions with each worksheet you complete. The same thoughts and emotions will likely recur. Mentally review the episode as soon afterward as possible. It is easier to catch the thoughts when they are "hot." If you are trying to figure them out later, try to imagine yourself in the actual situation.

Questioning Automatic Thoughts

Do some of your automatic thoughts seem silly when you review them? This is quite normal. Many thoughts seem silly in retrospect. In his practice, Dr. Claiborn often tells a story about one of his children in order to illustrate where some of these thoughts come from. Years ago, when she was just a little girl, his daughter liked to run under the lawn sprinkler in her bathing suit on hot days. She was doing this one day, when she realized she needed to go to the bathroom. She couldn't remove her bathing suit because a knot behind her neck held it fastened, and she had trouble reaching the knot. She came running to her father and started to cry, sure that she would *never, ever* get the bathing suit off. He was able to help her untie the knot, however, in plenty of time for her to get to the bathroom.

This is an illustration of one of the ways children think. Dr. Claiborn's daughter believed that if she could not solve the problem right away then there would be no way to solve it—*ever*. This thought was upsetting to her. Unlike adults, young children say aloud the things they are thinking. We may laugh at the things they say, but we understand that this type of thinking, sometimes distorted or irrational, is appropriate in a child. As we grow up, our childhood beliefs don't always go away. They can become automatic thoughts in many situations. We don't often say them aloud, but they remain in our minds. This is why we often get upset about little events that, when we look at them later, are really not important or logical things to be upset about. Many of the automatic thoughts and beliefs about appearance reflect things we have been told or heard repeated around us. For example, advertisements and mass media, which bombard us with images and messages about what looks good and how important it is to look good, can contribute to our automatic thoughts (see chapters 2 and 3).

When people first start recording their automatic thoughts they are often embarrassed to show them to anyone else, even their therapists. If you feel embarrassed, understand that we all think in irrational, childlike ways much of the time. Usually these thinking patterns are just fine since many of the simple rules we learned as children work in most situations. If we are doing something more complex, however, we may have to slow down and use more rational, adult ways of thinking. In the rest of this chapter and in the next one, we will look at how you can begin changing the patterns of thinking that make up your automatic thoughts. It is not necessary to try to change all, or even most, of your automatic thoughts, but it is important to change the thoughts in those areas of your life where they are causing problems.

Now let's take a closer look at why some of these *problem automatic thoughts* are so upsetting. We will begin with some thoughts that Casey had. After breast augmentation surgery, Casey felt more attractive and confident for a few weeks, but then she began to obsess about the shapes of her breasts. When she looked at herself in the mirror, she saw lumpy, deformed breasts. She wrote down the following thoughts. "I look awful. I should not go out in public because I am so unattractive. Everyone who sees me will think I am repulsive. My husband will be horribly ashamed and disgusted with me. I'm a terrible person. I just want to die or disappear." These automatic thoughts are typical of what someone with BDD might think and are perhaps somewhat harsher than but similar to the thoughts of someone with a less severe body-image problem. Next we will look at some of these thoughts a little more carefully, so we can understand what is going on.

- *"My husband will be horribly ashamed and disgusted with me."* Here, Casey seems to be engaging in some sort of mind-reading exercise. She is making *predictions* about how others (in this case her husband) will react when they look at her. Automatic thoughts that make predictions come in several forms, including mind reading, making predictions about your future, and assuming how you will feel at some future time. While it is reasonable and sometimes important to make some guesses about the future and some types of predictions about how others will act or think, it is important to keep in mind that no one has the ability to really predict these things. People with body-image problems often make predictions about how others will see them and what others will find appealing or attractive. Researchers have shown that men with muscle dysmorphia BDD predict that women will find a very muscular body more attractive, when women's actual preferences are for much more ordinary body types (Pope, Phillips, and Olivandria 2000).

- *"I look awful ... I look so repulsive."* Casey thinks that she looks awful and repulsive. These statements are conclusions. One of the most interesting things about these types of conclusions is that they are not based on any evidence, but rather on a "feeling." This type of thinking ("I am repulsive because I feel I am repulsive") has been called emotional reasoning. It's important to stop and examine the evidence for these conclusions. Let's think about conclusions as possible *problem automatic thoughts*. What happens if we just accept conclusions (our own or other people's) without asking some questions? We may find ourselves in trouble.

The statement "The world is flat" is a conclusion. If it were correct, Columbus would have sailed off of the edge of the world. We have lots of evidence that this conclusion is not true. In fact, even though you probably haven't tested the idea yourself, you would likely judge the conclusion that the world is flat to be silly. Suppose you came up with an *alternative conclusion*, one more in line with the evidence, such as "The world sometimes appears to be flat, but scientists say it is not." You could do the same thing with your thoughts about your body. How would that change the way you feel? For example, Casey might think, "Even though I feel that I look repulsive, no one really treats me that way, so maybe I look passable. My husband usually says I look fine, so he may even believe this." Arriving at these conclusions might lead to your being much less distressed when you go out in public.

- **"I should not go out in public because I am so gross looking."** This is a "should" statement. "Should" statements are a problem, partly because they are absolute statements. If you really think about it, there are very few absolutes in life and we need to be skeptical when they come up. We need to look for evidence that supports "should" statement, just as we want to do when looking at conclusions. A "should" statement implies that there is a rule or law that covers the situation. It is like a commandment: "Thou shalt not go out in public if you look awful." But where does that commandment come from? Is there such a rule or law at all? Would you tell anyone else to live by that rule? We don't think you will find that rule or law anywhere but in your own thoughts. People seem to make up these rules for themselves as they go along, often *after* they have broken them.

  When you run across a "should" statement, ask yourself some questions: Does this involve a moral law or a legal statute? Is it really just a good idea? Then that is not the same as a law. Can you rephrase it so it is not an absolute rule? For example, what would happen if you said to yourself, "I would rather not go out when I feel bad about how I look." It may change things somewhat to realize that you might be uncomfortable but you are not breaking some ironclad rule. This simple change in the thought tends to make "should" statements much less upsetting.

  Duncan, who picked at his skin, also seemed to be ruled by "should" statements in his automatic thoughts: "I should not pick my skin." He could change this to "I would look better if I didn't pick my skin." As you can see, the alternative thoughts can be much less upsetting than "should" statements. The should statements don't change anything that has already happened or help us learn anything new, but they do cause anxiety and stress.

- **"I just want to die or disappear."** This is really a *problem-solving thought*. Casey is thinking of some way to make herself feel better. Problem-solving thoughts in this type of situation might also include statements such as, "I will find an outfit that hides the way I look." While this idea may help temporarily solve her problem it is really working against her, because she is accepting the problem as legitimate in the first place. Problem-solving thoughts can be part of the problem or part of the solution. What makes the difference is what conclusions you started with.

Take a look at your Body-Image-Related Behaviors, Thoughts, and Emotions worksheets. Can you find any predictions, conclusions, or "should" statements? If you are like most people, you will find some of the same automatic thoughts showing up repeatedly. Make seven copies of the blank Alternative Body-Image Thoughts worksheet, which follows. Then complete the worksheet. List as many problem automatic thoughts as you can find. Then write down evidence to support the automatic thoughts and conclusions. Finally, write down these thoughts with alternative thoughts that are supported by the evidence. Complete one of these worksheets every day for the next week. We have provided an example of Alfred's Alternative Body-Image Thoughts.

As you can see, predictions, conclusions, and "should" statements can cause a great deal of anxiety and stress. They can also help us justify and rationalize counterproductive behavior. Replacing them with more realistic alternative thoughts can remove some of the justifications that perpetuate your negative body image. Notice that the alternative thoughts don't invalidate how you feel but they do help you put it into perspective. We are not criticizing the way you feel; we are only saying that feelings are not the same as facts. It is important to look at your conclusions and see if there is evidence to support them—are they based on feelings or facts?

Learning to catch automatic thoughts and develop alternatives is hard work. You may have trouble doing it and may reach the conclusion that you can't do it or that it won't help. However, these are just more automatic thoughts that come with some of the same problems. The idea that you can't do it is a conclusion made without evidence. A more realistic alternative would be, "This is a hard thing to learn and I am having trouble. If I continue to practice it I will probably gradually get better at it." The thought that it won't help is a prediction. How do you know it won't help? An alternative thought might be, "The experts seem to think this kind of thing helps people, so I could keep trying it and see if it helps me."

In this chapter we have started to look at how your thoughts and emotions are connected and how you can begin to modify them. In the next chapter we will work on some additional ways of looking at thoughts and how to change them. We will also look at the underlying core beliefs that contribute to your body-image problem.

 Image Balancing Strategy

As you listen to your automatic thoughts, consider what you would tell a friend, and talk to yourself as you would to a friend. Be your own best friend.

Alternative Body Image Thoughts

Problem Thought	Evidence and Arguments to Change the Thought	Alternative Thought

Alfred's Alternative Body Image Thoughts

Problem Thought	Evidence and Arguments to Change the Thought	Alternative Thought
My body is disgusting.	I think my arms are too small and misshapen, but that doesn't mean they actually are. That is my opinion. My arms don't define my entire body.	I feel as if my body is disgusting because, in my opinion, my arms are too small and misshapen. A feeling is not a fact.
I need to make my arms bigger.	Who says my arms need to be bigger?	I would like my arms to be bigger. They may be acceptable as they are.
I should eat more and exercise more so my arms will be bigger.	My arms don't define my entire body. If I eat more and gain weight, will that be good for my health?	Eating more and exercising may make them bigger. But doing things like that in the past has not made me feel much better.
I'm disgusting.	Even if my body is disgusting, does that make me disgusting?	I feel disgusting. Feelings aren't facts. I am acceptable.
I can't go out looking like this. People will stare and I'll be embarrassed.	Who's stopping me from going out? How do I know for sure that people will stare? How do I know they are staring at me? If they do stare, if I'm convinced that they are staring, that doesn't mean I have to be embarrassed.	I prefer not to go out when I don't feel like I look good. People might stare and that might make me feel like they are staring at my arms. People may not be looking at me as much as I think they are. I can't know what they think.

CHAPTER 9

Mindfully Challenging Core Beliefs about Body Image

n the last chapter, we looked at how your ways of thinking can be connected to emotional distress and how changing your thinking habits can help you change how distressed you are. Let's explore other ways to change thoughts that are destructive to your body image.

Facilitating Thoughts

Allison was contemplating taking diet pills, exercising to excess, vomiting after meals, or smoking to lose weight. She had some particular thoughts and beliefs that made it more likely that she would engage in these actions. For example, she believed that she needed to be thinner in order to be liked and respected. Similarly, Brad was tempted to use anabolic steroids to build muscles and make his body look like those shown in bodybuilding magazines. He believed he should strive for perfection in his appearance or else be seen as weak and repulsive. Think of these as *facilitating thoughts*. If Brad accepts them as valid his decision to take steroids or engage in other appearance-changing behaviors is facilitated or encouraged.

Facilitating thoughts include the permission-giving thoughts we discussed in chapter 8. They are born of beliefs we hold before we are faced with a trigger situation. It is important to understand how these thoughts work. There's an old joke about a man who whistled all the time. When his friends asked him why he whistled so much, his answer was that it kept man-eating tigers away. His friends would say, "There are no man-eating tigers for thousands of miles." The man would reply, "It works pretty well, doesn't it?" Facilitating thoughts can lead to behaviors such as avoiding going out, wearing special clothes, or spending hours fixing your appearance. Like whistling to keep tigers away, not having the feared experience is attributed to all these efforts. You become convinced that you need to engage in the behavior.

What kind of facilitating thoughts keep you engaged in appearance-related rituals? Spotting these automatic facilitating thoughts can be difficult at first, so below we've listed facilitating thoughts for Morgan, who was overly concerned about the dark circles under her eyes. For each facilitating thought, develop a more reasonable thought. We've provided space for one of each, but you'll probably find many more over time. Make a collection of facilitating thoughts and their more reasonable alternatives. It might help to print these on three-by-five-inch cards and tape them up in places where you'll likely run into trigger situations.

Facilitating thought: _____

Reasonable thought: _____

Morgan: **Facilitating thought:** *I will look acceptable if I lighten the dark areas under my eyes. I can find a cream that will make this look okay.*

Morgan: **Reasonable thought:** *It is part of my normal appearance to have dark circles under my eyes. Even if some people think I look tired it would not be the end of the world.*

Distorted Thoughts

The thoughts that are causing us problems are based on beliefs, including some we don't acknowledge consciously. Often, we just haven't paid attention to them or examined them to see if they are valid or reasonable. In chapter 8, we discussed predictions, "should" statements, and conclusions. These are all automatic thoughts that are based on some of our underlying core beliefs. Remember the diagram below showing how events lead to automatic thoughts, which in turn lead to emotional reactions?

Events   →   Automatic thoughts   →   Emotional reaction

↑

Core beliefs

Both the automatic thoughts and the core beliefs can be, and frequently are, distorted in one way or another. Let's examine how these thoughts and beliefs may be distorted and look at some ways to identify and even change them. Remember the story about Dr. Claiborn's daughter and the bathing suit? That was an example of distorted thinking. We thought in distorted ways as children because, with our limited life experience, that is how we understood the world around us. We also developed our core beliefs when we were children. Many of us don't change our core beliefs or the way we think when we grow up, however, and the patterns become automatic. Everyone, regardless of education, intelligence, age, or social status, has some distorted automatic thoughts.

We are not telling you that you are bad or wrong for having distorted thoughts. We are suggesting that some of these thoughts may lead to the behaviors that you use to reduce your distress. Like whistling to keep tigers away, however, your efforts to make yourself feel better only serve as temporary relief and end up persuading you that you did indeed need to do them. The diagram below demonstrates this progression of thoughts and behaviors.

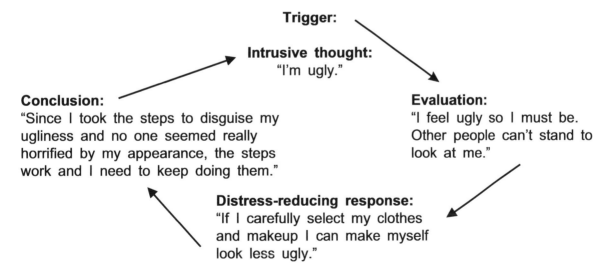

Trigger:

Intrusive thought:
"I'm ugly."

Evaluation:
"I feel ugly so I must be. Other people can't stand to look at me."

Distress-reducing response:
"If I carefully select my clothes and makeup I can make myself look less ugly."

Conclusion:
"Since I took the steps to disguise my ugliness and no one seemed really horrified by my appearance, the steps work and I need to keep doing them."

As you can see from this diagram, efforts to make yourself look better or reduce your distress over appearance really only provide temporary relief and lead to a vicious circle of intrusive thoughts and efforts to make yourself feel better.

Sometimes you may attempt to make yourself feel better by trying to control or prevent the intrusive thoughts in the first place. This leads to an increase in the thoughts and may make you feel even more powerless. Dr. Claiborn teaches people about these obsessive thoughts by doing a little experiment that you can try now. Think about polar bears for one minute. When you find your mind wandering, go back to thinking about polar bears. You probably had some non-bear-related thoughts but could bring yourself back to thinking about the bears quickly and easily. The next part of the experiment is much harder. For the next one minute, *don't* think about polar bears at all. Try as hard as you can *not* to think about polar bears. Almost everyone will find that they cannot keep themselves from thinking about polar bears. This can be a little amusing and in general is not upsetting. However, when you have an intrusive thought that *is* upsetting, such as "My cheeks are red like a clown's and I look like a child," you may find it very upsetting. When you try not to have that thought, it comes into mind even more. The more upset you get, the more you try to push it out of your mind, and the more it pops up. Other, distorted thoughts, such as "I should be able to control my thoughts," or "If I have a thought it must be important and true," may appear and make you more upset.

Dr. David Burns has written several good self-help books, listed in the Resources section of this book, that use a cognitive approach to helping people understand their thinking and the distortions in it. In *The Feeling Good Handbook* (1990), Dr. Burns lists ten distortions that show up in most people's thinking. He helps readers to first identify the distortions in their own thinking, then learn to think in a less distorted fashion. Other authors including Dr. Albert Ellis and Dr. Aaron Beck have developed similar lists. Many of the individual distortions included in these lists overlap. We've narrowed them down to three—*drawing conclusions without evidence, thinking in absolute terms,* and *making predictions.* We believe these three types of thought distortions represent the major problems for people with body-image problems.

Drawing Conclusions without Evidence

We discussed drawing conclusions without evidence in chapter 8. If you are familiar with Dr. Burns's list of distortions, you may understand drawing conclusions without evidence to include *jumping to conclusions, discounting the positive, magnification, minimization, blame, mental filtering,* and *emotional reasoning.* All of these distortions have one thing in common—we arrive at a conclusion about ourselves or the rest of the world without evaluating the data.

Mental filtering is a process in which we selectively pay attention only to data that supports our ideas without evaluating the rest of the information. This process is involved in discounting the positive, magnification, minimization, and blame.

Emotional reasoning means thinking, "I feel this way, so it must be true." This use of feelings as evidence is a problem since it really represents arriving at a conclusion, then using the conclusion as evidence to support itself. For example, "I feel ugly, therefore I must be ugly. How do I know it's true? Because I feel that way." An effective method for dealing with these thoughts begins with the recognition that we are drawing a conclusion without evaluating evidence. Then if we evaluate the thought in a nondistorted way and remember that feelings, no matter how strong, are not facts, we may arrive at a different conclusion. For example, it might be accurate to say, "I feel ugly, but I have no evidence to show that others think so or that it affects how they treat me, so perhaps the feeling is not that important." A feeling is not a fact.

Thinking in Absolute Terms

In chapter 8, we discussed "should" statements. The basic problem with these is that they are absolute. Dr. Burns includes other distortions in his list that are examples of absolute thinking—*all-or-nothing thinking, labeling,* and *overgeneralization.*

All-or-nothing thinking is usually involved in perfectionism. You may think of yourself as falling into one of two absolute categories: beautiful or ugly; thin or fat. This type of thinking creates a problem when you are trying to change problem habits associated with body-image dissatisfaction. You might think, "I am a skin picker and I can't ever control myself," "If I start I have to finish," or "If I am going to fix my hair I have to do it until I am satisfied, no matter how long it takes." An example of labeling is "If my arms are too skinny, then I am a weakling and a failure." Calling yourself a weakling or a failure is putting yourself into an absolute category. We might ask, weak compared to whom? Have you failed at everything in life or simply in getting the appearance you want? Overgeneralization involves seeing negative events as part of a never-ending or absolute pattern: "It will never get better." This particular thought often occurs in people who are depressed. It may be expressed by someone with a body-image problem in this way: "That person looked away when I walked in, so that means everyone is bothered by my appearance."

The problem with absolute thoughts is that they usually don't fit what's happening in the real world. In reality there are a few absolutes, but they are rare, and most of us don't encounter them very often. One way to counteract problem absolute thoughts is to ask yourself if you can think of an exception. If you can, then you can try to come up with an alternative thought that is not absolute but does fit the evidence and data you have. Arnold thought his red cheeks and small eyes made him look like a clown and seem childish. He believed everyone would treat him like a child or a clown. But when he thought about his everyday interactions with other people, he could see that most of the time people did not seem to pay much attention to his cheeks at all and that most people seemed to treat him in the same way they treated everybody else.

Making Predictions

The third type of thought distortion that is a source of trouble for many people with body-image problems is making predictions. Most anxiety really comes from making predictions. Dr. Burns writes about mind reading and fortune telling, which are examples of this type of distortion. A common form of prediction is the "what if?" thought. This often occurs when people think about how others will see them. You might think, "What if they see how ugly I am?" and then mentally answer this by making a prediction, "They will see that I am ugly and distorted and want me to go away. They will be repulsed and sickened." This type of prediction may seem silly to someone else, but when it is your own you will likely take it quite seriously.

We often make predictions about not being able to handle things, or about facing impossible obstacles: "I will be so embarrassed I will just die." Another form of prediction is the "I can't stand" statement. You may think, "I can't stand to leave this one blemish alone," or "I can't stand to have this distorted face." Ask yourself what it means to not be able to stand something. The famous psychologist Albert Ellis says, "You can stand anything, including being run over by a steam roller, until it kills you. Then you don't have to stand it anymore." When we say we can't stand something, we are really making a prediction about what will happen if we try. The fact is that, in most cases, we will be uncomfortable, perhaps even extremely uncomfortable, but we can stand it and may have no choice.

In chapter 8, we also talked about permission giving thoughts. These thoughts often come with their own predictions (for example, "If I build up muscles enough, I will look and feel better."). The best way to deal with prediction distortions is to use the three-question technique. Ask yourself three critical questions.

1. What exactly am I predicting?

2. What is the probability of that prediction coming true?

3. If it did come true, what would the consequences be?

Write these questions on a three-by-five-inch card and carry it with you. When you find yourself making predictions, pull out the card and answer the questions for yourself. Alfred predicted, "Everyone will stare at my arms." He predicted the probability was 25 percent, and that the consequences would be that "Those people might think I have scrawny arms." Answering these questions helped him put his fears into perspective.

The following Distorted Thought Record (DTR) will help you examine your automatic thoughts to identify distortions. It is like the Alternative Body-Image Thoughts chart you completed in chapter 8, but it takes the process much further and will help you gain a better understanding of how your thoughts about your appearance may be distorted. In the first column, describe a situation or train of thought that triggered your body-image concerns. In the second column, in a few words, describe how you were feeling. Then, in the third column, record your automatic thoughts. You may have quite a few, but the most important ones are those that are connected to your emotional response and those that are involved in facilitating the behaviors you use to reduce your distress. In the fourth column, identify the distortions in your thoughts. Label them using the categories we described: conclusions without evidence, absolute statements, and predictions. In the last column, record the evidence you have for the automatic thoughts, along with an alternative automatic thought. Write the evidence supporting the alternative thought as well. We've provided Alfred's DTR as an example. Notice how the alternative thought is likely to lead to a different emotional reaction.

Core Beliefs

Next, we need to understand the core beliefs that can cause problems. Everyone has their own set of core beliefs. Some of these beliefs can be quite distorted and can cause great distress. Many of these core beliefs are ones we learned early in life and are never spoken about or even acknowledged. One way of understanding core beliefs is to consider them as a kind of template or mold that we use to shape our automatic thoughts. For example, if you have a core belief that your worth is based on what others think of you, automatic thoughts such as, "If I don't look good I am worthless" will be likely to pop into your head. The thought is a specific example or extension of the more basic belief.

Since core beliefs serve as templates for our automatic thoughts, it is important to identify them and, when they are distorted, to attempt to modify them. One of the best ways to identify core beliefs is to use a flowchart. Start with an upsetting automatic thought and ask yourself, "If this thought were true, what would it mean?" Keep asking

Distorted Thought Record

Situation	Emotional Reaction	Automatic Thought	Type of Distortion	Review of Evidence and Alternative Thought

Alfred's Distorted Thought Record

Situation	Emotional Reaction	Automatic Thought	Type of Distortion	Review of Evidence and Alternative Thought
Getting dressed to go to the gym.	Disgust, anxiety.	I look horrible. My arms are scrawny looking.	Conclusion	My arms are *so* thin. They are thinner than some people's, but they are bigger than others.
At the gym, trying to concentrate on working out.	Anxiety, racing thoughts.	I just have to gain more muscle so I won't look so weak and disgusting.	Absolute	I would like to gain more muscle. But will that make me look less weak or be less weak? Even after I gain some weight, I might still feel like I look weak.
Looking around me and noticing other people looking at me.	Anxiety, disgusted, fear.	They are looking at me, probably at my arms. Even in long sleeves, my arms look hideous.	Conclusion	Those people appear to be looking at me. They might be looking at someone else or they might be noticing something else about me. I have no proof that they are even noticing my arms.
Weighing myself at the gym.	Disappointment	I eat and eat, and still I don't gain weight. If only I weighed more my arms would look better and I wouldn't look so disgusting.	Prediction	If I gain weight, I might still feel like I look disgusting. Perhaps I could base my eating and exercise decisions on overall health instead.
At home, looking in mirror, trying to decide if I dare go to a movie.	Depression, fatigue.	I'd like to go to a movie, but I might run into someone I know. I just couldn't stand someone seeing me until I can get my arms looking better.	Prediction	If I go out someone I know might see me. Even if they react negatively, I could probably stand it. I can handle it. How long can I put off going out in public? If I wait until I feel like I look okay, that day may never come.

Chart 9b

until you find a basic belief that forms or shapes the automatic thought. Alfred used an automatic thought from his Distorted Thought Record.

Alfred's automatic thought: *My arms are scrawny looking.*

↓

If that statement were true, it would mean: *Everyone will see how scrawny and ugly they are.*

↓

If that statement were true, it would mean: *Everyone will see what a worthless, ugly person I am.*

↓

If that statement were true, it would mean: *I am a worthless person.*

The core belief that he is a worthless person is causing Alfred a great deal of distress. Believing he is worthless may lead him to get more depressed and give up on life. He may stop going out at all because it seems so hopeless and he feels so helpless. Pick one of your automatic thoughts and try to discover the basic belief behind it.

Automatic thought:

↓

If that statement were true, it would mean:

↓

If that statement were true, it would mean:

↓

If that statement were true, it would mean:

Once you've discovered some of your problem core beliefs, it is important that you challenge them and work on changing them. Look for the evidence. If you can't find evidence to support the belief, form a more reasonable alternative belief. The Problem Belief Challenge worksheet will help you do this. At the top of the first column, write the basic belief you found by completing the flowchart above. Write an alternative, or revised, belief at the top of the next column. During the next week, list the evidence you gather each day that supports the core belief and evidence that supports the alternative belief. We've provided Alfred's Problem Belief Challenge worksheet as an example. We recommend keeping this kind of record on a regular basis while you are actively trying to work on your body-image problem. Because these beliefs are active in a range of situations that upset you or leave you feeling bad, using this method to change your core beliefs to more reasonable ones will help you improve many areas of your life, not only your body-image problem.

You may also find behavioral experiments helpful in changing core beliefs. We describe these in some detail in chapter 13.

Mindfulness and Disgust

One interesting thing about BDD and related disorders is that many people seem to react with disgust to their perceived defect, in addition to or instead of anxiety. This is true of OCD and phobias, as well as BDD. Anxiety habituates to exposure; when we are repeatedly exposed to the things that cause anxiety and don't engage in our distress-reducing behaviors that make us feel better, the anxiety fades and we learn to respond with much less distress to our triggers for anxiety. This is the result of a change in the evaluation of the intrusive thoughts. But what happens if an intrusive thought is evaluated in a way that leads to disgust instead of anxiety? Disgust is like anxiety in that it seems to be a basic emotional response built into each of us. However, it may not respond in exactly the same way to exposure as anxiety does.

Only a little research on disgust has been done so far, but disgust seems to be different from anxiety in how it habituates. It also appears to be more directly tied to those core beliefs we discussed earlier. You can have a lot of anxiety about something, but you're more likely to see it as outside yourself so the anxiety doesn't connect to a core belief about yourself. A disgust response about yourself, however, would connect to your core beliefs about yourself. Suppose someone has a spider phobia—he or she thinks that spiders are disgusting and avoids them at all costs. Spiders are thought of as the bad thing. If you think your nose is horrible and ugly, and you avoid looking at it or letting anyone else see it, you are thinking of yourself as disgusting.

We can use our knowledge of OCD to help us understand how we can work with this disgust problem. People with BDD and people with OCD both have upsetting thoughts. There are important differences in the content of the thoughts, but the experience is similar. The obsessive thoughts of OCD center on such fears as harm coming to self or others. People with OCD often evaluate the thoughts as important and meaning something about themselves, perhaps that there is something horrible about a person who would have such thoughts. In BDD, thoughts involves the idea that there is something horrible about the person's appearance. Researchers have studied these intrusive thoughts in OCD. They have found that everyone, not just people with OCD, has them. This tells us that it is not the occurrence of the thought that causes a problem, but the evaluation of the thoughts. For example, if someone has a thought about harming someone else, we know the thought is not unusual and that it doesn't mean anything about the person having it. However, if he or she evaluates the thought, thinks it is important, pays attention to it, or tries to force the thought out of mind, this creates distress.

Remember the polar bears? The same principle applies here. Everyone has negative thoughts about some aspect of their appearance. Dr. Claiborn will admit that he has a stomach that's too big and hair that's too thin for his liking. However, when these thoughts come to mind, he accepts that he is not perfect, or even especially good looking, but does not pass further judgment. It is in situations like this that we need to remember to be mindful. Turn your evaluation into nonjudgmental acceptance of the occurrence of the thought. Remember that the thought is no more important than the random thoughts about polar bears you had earlier; it simply needs to be observed and experienced, and finally allowed to pass from your mind. If the thought occurs to you that you have a horribly deformed nose, accept that such thoughts tend to occur, as evidenced by the fact that it just occurred to you. The thought is no more important than the random thoughts you had about polar bears earlier in this chapter. Any experience or thought is only as important as you make it. Observe it, accept it, and do not devote time or energy to evaluating it; simply experience it. This mindful way of responding means that you are not engaging the negative core belief. You are recognizing negative thoughts and mindfully deciding how to treat them, rather than automatically taking them to their usual negative conclusions.

This and the preceding chapter have focused on changing the way you think. Changing the way you think changes the way you feel, helps relieve depression and anxiety, and changes the importance you give to body image. It is important to remember that thinking involves habits. Much of this book is about changing habits. You can use ideas described in other parts of the book, such as the competing response (see chapter 11), relaxation, and mindfulness to help change your thinking habits. Keep this in mind as we now go on to changing body-image-related behavior. You may need to come back to these chapters while you are working on your body-image problem and repeat the exercises. Changing the way you think is hard work, but it can be done.

Problem Belief Challenge

Day	Original Basic Belief: _____ _____ Evidence That Supports the Belief	Revised Basic Belief: _____ _____ Evidence That Supports the Belief
1		
2		
3		
4		
5		
6		
7		

Chart 9c

Alfred's Problem Belief Challenge

Day	Original Basic Belief: *I am a worthless person.* **Evidence That Supports the Belief**	Revised Basic Belief: *I am a person of value* **Evidence That Supports the Belief**
1	I am disgusted with the way my arms look.	I am kind to other people.
2	I lost a pound. I can't even eat enough to keep weight on.	I have eaten a healthy diet today.
3	No one paid attention to me when I went to the store. They were probably avoiding me.	I avoided eye contact so no one had reason to interact with me.
4	My sister asked me why I always wear long sleeves. She thinks I'm weird.	My sister might be concerned about me. Perhaps she is worried. She cares.
5	I stayed home today because going out seemed too distressing.	My dad called to see how I was.
6	My shoulders are sore from holding my arms in certain positions so they look better, but still I can't get them to look right.	My shoulders felt better after I did my relaxation exercises. I also didn't feel quite as concerned about my arms and noticed that my hair was looking nice today.
7	I looked at a bodybuilding magazine and felt worse than ever. I'll never look like any of those guys.	My cat reminded me it was time for dinner. I'm really important to him.

Chart 9d

CHAPTER 10

Changing Body-Image-Related Behaviors through Exposure and Response Prevention

You have been learning to change negative, self-defeating thoughts through time-tested cognitive behavioral therapy techniques. Now, we'll help you attack your self-defeating behaviors. You've already started to change your behavior by practicing daily relaxation techniques. This is your opportunity to treat your body and your mind in a positive way. Relaxation will become even more important to you as you make some major changes in your body-image-related behaviors. In making these changes, we will utilize two powerful behavior therapy techniques: exposure and response prevention, and habit reversal.

Exposure and Response Prevention

Exposure and response prevention (ERP) involves exposing yourself to situations you fear and preventing yourself from responding in your usual self-defeating manner. For our purposes, a better term for this technique might be exposure and response *change*. You won't be preventing a response; you will be changing your usual response. After all, even doing nothing is a response.

Review your Self-Image Journals. When faced with obsessive thoughts, worries, and body-image concerns, you learned to respond in certain ways. At first, these behaviors temporarily relieved your anxiety and distress. The key word here is *temporarily*. At first, the responses helped, but the relief didn't last and the anxiety returned, perhaps worse than before. These behaviors keep the cycle going. Preventing your usual response, or changing your response, can break the cycle and reduce the obsessive thoughts about your body.

The first step is to determine what situations make you more likely to have obsessive thoughts, worries, body-image concerns, and self-defeating behaviors. In what circumstances are you the most anxious about your appearance? What activities and situations do you avoid? Are your body-image concerns the worst at social events? Do you avoid looking at yourself in the mirror? Or do you compulsively check your image in the mirror? Do dressing, applying makeup, or bathing make you feel worse about your body image? Do these activities trigger compulsive behaviors, such as checking, changing clothes, or skin picking? Do these same activities increase your negative thoughts? These are the types of situations you will put on your Stressful Situations List.

Over the course of several days, list all the situations or activities that increase your anxiety about your appearance. Continue the list on a separate piece of paper if you run out of room. When you've completed your list, rank each situation or activity by the level of anxiety it provokes. We'll use the Subjective Units of Distress Scale (SUDS), a method of self-rating anxiety developed by Joseph Wolpe, M.D., at Temple University to express the levels of distress associated with each situation or activity. SUDS is a 100-point scale, with 0 equaling no anxiety at all and 100 equaling extreme anxiety. We've provided Leo's Stressful Situations List as an example. Leo, who wanted everything to be in order and combed and trimmed his hair compulsively, was diagnosed with obsessive-compulsive disorder and body dysmorphic disorder.

Stressful Situations List

Situation or Activity	SUDS Level 0–100

Leo's Stressful Situations List

Situation or Activity	SUDS Level 0–100
Getting ready to go to the mall and spending only 10 minutes on my hair.	*40*
Going to the mall and not checking my hair after leaving the house.	*45*
Getting ready for work and spending only 10 minutes on my hair.	*50*
Going to a meeting at work without checking my hair first.	*60*
Getting ready to go out with family or friends and spending only 10 minutes on my hair.	*50*
Going out with family or friends and not checking my hair after leaving the house.	*60*
Getting ready for a social event and spending only 10 minutes on my hair.	*80*
Going to a social event where women are present and not checking my hair after leaving the house.	*90*
Getting a haircut without checking and trimming my hair or side-burns afterward.	*95*
Giving away my pocket mirror.	*100*

Chart 10b

Behavioral Responses

When you are faced with situations that trigger body-image dissatisfaction, what do you do? Do you avoid the situations or activities? Or do you respond with compulsive behavior, such as checking, changing clothes, seeking reassurance, skin picking, hair pulling, or comparing yourself with models? At first, these responses probably temporarily relieved some of your anxiety. But now, they have become compulsive. Your responses to body-image dissatisfaction fall into two categories—compulsive responses and avoidance responses. List these responses in the following worksheets. Review your Self-Image Journal to find responses you might not otherwise remember. Rate each response by the frequency with which you engage in it, according to the following scale:

1 = rarely
2 = occasionally
3 = often
4 = very often

We've provided Leo's Compulsive Response and Avoidance Response worksheets as examples. You might put some responses on both charts, as Leo did with "getting a haircut." He got haircuts with the hope of having the stylist even his hair, but he also avoided getting haircuts because he knew he would spend days checking and trimming his hair and sideburns afterward.

Response Changes

You've collected some valuable information. You've identified the situations and activities in which you are most dissatisfied with your body image and you've described your usual response to these situations and activities. The next step is to change the response. But, you may be saying, that would cause anxiety! Yes it would, but that is part of the goal of ERP. When you deliberately expose yourself to scary situations without engaging in your usual response to relieve the distress, you will experience distress, anxiety, worry, or disgust. When Leo thought his hair or sideburns were uneven, he didn't just feel some uneasiness, he felt disgusted with his appearance and great embarrassment. However, repeated exposure will reduce your distress, you'll begin to realize that the outcome isn't as bad as you thought it would be, and that you can indeed handle the anxiety.

If you were to start with a situation or activity with the highest SUDS score on your list of stressful situations, you would soon become discouraged. Instead choose a situation with a moderate score, one that causes only moderate distress. Leo started with getting ready for work, which he had given a SUDS of 50. He felt that he might be able to handle it. He also felt that exposure to this activity would help him the most because his BDD was having a great effect on his work.

With each situation or activity, you will change your response. Your new response needs to be one that takes the focus off of your body image, one that doesn't seek correction of or reassurance about your perceived defect—a more balanced response. Essentially, you need to do what you fear. There are a variety of ways to change your responses. We've listed some below.

- **Don't engage in any response.** This may be the best solution, but if it seems to be too anxiety provoking, try one of the other responses at first.

Compulsive Responses

Behavior	Frequency

Leo's Compulsive Responses

Behavior	Frequency
Check hair in bathroom mirror.	4
Check hair in pocket mirror.	3
Check hair in visor mirror in car.	3
Comb and re-comb hair.	4
Look at other people's hair and sideburns to see if theirs are even.	2
Trim hair or sideburns in bathroom.	3
Trim hair or sideburns with scissors in car, looking in the visor mirror.	3
Trim hair or sideburns with manicure scissors that I keep in my desk drawer at work.	2
Wash hair 2 to 3 times a day, sometimes more.	4
Wear hat to hide hair.	3
Pat hair with hands.	4
Get unneeded hair cut.	2
Apply excessive mousse, gel, hair spray.	4
Purchase new hair products.	3
Ask for other people's opinion about my hair.	4
Look at the hair and sideburns of models in magazines and on TV.	2
Check hair in windows of stores as I'm walking by.	3
Check hair in mirrors, at home, in restrooms, anywhere there is a mirror.	4

Chart 10d

Avoidance Responses

Avoided Activities or Situations	Frequency

Chart 10e

Leo's Avoidance Responses

Avoided Activities or Situations	Frequency
Going to social events	4
Going to work	2
Going to meetings at work	3
Going to lunch with friends	3
Getting haircuts	3
Getting together with friends and family	3
Going to church	2
Being seen under bright lights and sunlight, where hair is more noticeable	3
Going to the mall, grocery store, or other stores	2
Being in wind and rain that can mess up my hair	4
Working out or doing other physical activities that would mess up my hair	4

Chart 10f

- **Change the response.** Change the way you respond to the situation. For example, you could exercise daily for twenty minutes instead of two hours.

- **Delay the response.** At first, you might find it too difficult to stop a compulsive behavior "cold turkey." Try delaying the behavior for a specific amount of time, then increasing the time gradually (not too gradually, though, because it is important to feel some anxiety).

- **Limit the response.** Some body-image-related behaviors are necessary but need to be limited. You need to get dressed, but you don't need to try on several outfits. You need to style your hair, but you don't need to spend an hour doing so. Use a timer or watch to limit your response.

- **Schedule your response.** Decide on a convenient time for the behavior and make an appointment with yourself. For example, you could plan to check your lipstick daily at 10:00 A.M. in the restroom at work. If you miss your appointment, wait until the next appointed time, say 11:30 A.M. Or you might plan to spend twenty minutes reading bodybuilding magazines every evening at 7:00 P.M. After a while, keeping the schedule might become such a nuisance that you forget your appointments altogether.

- **Replace the response.** Substitute the problem behavior with a new one. Here's a good rule of thumb: Do the opposite of what you are tempted to do. If you are avoiding looking at yourself in the mirror, then look at yourself. If you are excessively checking your appearance in the mirror, then avoid mirrors.

- **Rearrange your environment.** Make it more convenient to respond in a more balanced way to body-image-related distress. Put scissors, tweezers, scales, and other facilitating objects out of reach.

- **Do what you fear.** Stop avoiding what you fear. Look in mirrors if you usually avoid them. Go to social events you have been avoiding.

But how do you know if your responses to situations are excessive or not? How do you decide how long is too long and how much is too much? If you are working with a therapist, he or she will be able to help you. If you are working through *The BDD Workbook* on your own, ask a support person to help you identify reasonable, balanced responses to your stressful situations. Don't, however, consult people who have body-image-related problems of their own. You might conduct your own investigation, or informal research study. Find out: How often do other people fix their makeup? How long do others exercise? How long does it take others to style their hair? Keep track of the results, then decide on a balanced response to your stressful situation. Common sense will be your biggest ally. If you suspect your response might be out of balance, it probably is. Ask yourself, "Why am I doing this?" If you are doing it to reduce anxiety, worries, or disgust, change the response. As you proceed, you will likely become more courageous with your changes.

Make copies of the Exposure and Response Change Plan, which follows, and complete one for each stressful situation you've identified. Start with a situation in the middle of your list. If that seems too frightening, start with the situation with your lowest SUDS rating. Or you may want to divide the situation into more manageable parts. For example, you could divide going to a social event into going to a social event with a close friend and going to a social event alone.

We have included a place for you to write in your "reward." Changing is hard work. Give yourself a reward for working toward having a more balanced body image. Your daily relaxation time is one reward. Schedule it to happen very soon after you do your ERP with your feared situation. Think of other things you can do to reward yourself for your work to develop a more balanced body image and response. Often, your reward will be a natural outcome of your changes—more time to do other things, for example. It's important to recognize these rewards as the advantages of change. After you've done the ERP, assess your SUDS rating again. If it isn't down significantly, at least 20 percent, repeat the ERP. We've included Leo's Exposure and Response Change Plan as an example. These plans can also be useful for people without BDD. Calvin and Linda didn't have BDD, but they benefited from ERP, Calvin for his excessive fear of going bald and Linda for her excessive concerns about her hair and skin.

Continue completing Exposure and Response Change Plans until you run out of situations to challenge yourself with. Then start over. Go back and do the ERP using the same situations until you have a significant reduction of your anxiety or distress related to each situation. The next chapter will introduce you to another behavior therapy technique, habit reversal, which will be helpful with particular behaviors that have become almost habitual.

Exposure and Response Change Plan

Date: _____ **Situation**: _____

_____

Fear, worry, or body-image concern: _____

_____

_____

Usual response: _____

_____

_____

More balanced response: _____

_____

_____

Reward: _____

_____

Automatic thoughts: _____

_____

_____

More balanced thoughts: _____

_____

_____

Beginning SUDS: _____ **Ending SUDS**: _____

Leo's Exposure and Response Change Plan

Date: _8-5-02_   **Situation:** _Getting ready for work and spending only 10 minutes on my hair_

Fear, worry, or body-image concern: _My hair won't look right. It won't lay flat and will be uneven. The hair on one side will be longer than on the other. My sideburns will be uneven._

Usual response: _Spend an hour or more combing and styling hair, checking for evenness, trimming sideburns and hair, applying gel and hair spray. Then starting over—washing, drying, and styling again._

More balanced response: _Wash hair in shower, dry hair, add gel, comb, spend 10 minutes styling and combing hair. No trimming of hair or sideburns._

Reward: _Sleep 15 minutes later. Read the paper in the remaining time._

Automatic thoughts: _My hair doesn't look right. I have to make it look right. It needs to lay flat and be even. I'm disgusting._

More balanced thoughts: _I would like to have nice-looking hair, but I know it can't always look perfect. This will have to do._

Beginning SUDS: _50_   **Ending SUDS:** _35_

Chart 10h

CHAPTER 11

Changing Body-Image-Related Habits Using Habit Reversal

A habit is an acquired behavior that is done often, is almost automatic, and is difficult to stop. Some of your body-image related behaviors have become habits. Your automatic thoughts can also be habits. Even as you develop a more balanced body image, these habits may remain. Changing these behaviors will help you maintain your more balanced body image.

Behaviors such as fixing your appearance only reinforce the idea that you don't look right. Checking your appearance in the mirror reminds you that you're not satisfied with your looks. Avoidance behaviors reinforce your belief that you are unacceptable or that the anticipated situation would be too anxiety provoking. Derogatory self-talk about your appearance influences your beliefs about yourself and your body image. All of these behaviors and thoughts can become habits. After a while, they can become a way of life, so much so that you don't even remember why you engage in them. Some habits, such as skin picking, hair pulling, and excessive exercising, can even be harmful.

Habit Reversal

In the 1970s, psychologists and researchers Nathan Azrin and Gregory Nunn developed a behavior modification procedure for changing unwanted habits, called *habit reversal*, which is still used today. Habit reversal will give you additional tools to help you change your responses to distress-causing situations. Numerous studies have shown that habit reversal is effective in treating tics, nervous habits, and stuttering, and that it is generally effective in changing a variety of behaviors, with lasting results (Miltenberger, Fuqua, and Woods 1998). Habit reversal includes awareness training, competing response training, and motivation procedures.

Step 1: Keep a Record of Your Habit

The purpose of record keeping is to discover when your habit seems to affect your life the most. Your Habit Record will tell you when you had the urge to engage in the habit, whether you engaged in it or not, how long the urge lasted, and the automatic thoughts and emotional reactions you had. Take a look at your Self-Image Journal and your Compulsive Responses chart. Do certain behaviors show up over and over, enough to be considered habits? Skin picking, checking, and excessive grooming behaviors are common in people with BDD, but there are many other possibilities. Choose one to work on first; this may be your most bothersome habit, but if that seems too overwhelming, choose a habit that is less bothersome. Make copies of the Habit Record and the Triggers and Consequences Record, and keep track of your habit for five to seven days.

You may notice that just keeping records brings about changes in your habit. For example, recording everything you eat usually leads to a change of eating habits. Because of this fact, record keeping is important in habit change; not only does it help you become aware of where you started and how much you have changed, but it also brings about change. We have provided Delia's Habit Record and Triggers and Consequences Record as examples. She identified hair pulling and plucking, skin picking, and eye-makeup application as behaviors that had become habitual. She chose to use habit reversal on her skin-picking habit first.

Habit Record

Date and Time	Type of Urge	Did You Give In? Duration of Urge	Emotion(s)	Automatic Thoughts

Chart 11a

Delia's Habit Record

Date and Time	Type of Urge	Did You Give In? Duration of Urge	Emotion(s)	Automatic Thoughts
8/2 7:00 A.M.	Pick blemishes on face	Yes—45 minutes	Disgust, anxiety, fear	I'm so ugly. These pimples look horrible. I think I can smooth this out and make it look better.
8/2 10:00 A.M.	Pick at cuticles	Yes—10 minutes	Anxiety, nervousness	There I go again, picking at my fingers.
8/2 3:00 P.M.	Pick at cuticles	No—20 minutes	Anxiety	I don't need to pick at these cuticles. Just let them stay rough.
8/2 7:00 P.M.	Pick at blemishes on face	Yes—45 minutes	Disgust, nervousness	I'll smooth this one spot and make it look better.
8/2 10:00 P.M	Pick at blemishes on face	Yes—90 minutes	Disgust, worry, anxiety, fear	I know I shouldn't pick, but I need to fix this one spot. And this spot.
8/3 8:00 A.M.	Pick at blemishes on face	Yes—40 minutes?	Disgust, worry, fear	I need to look right today. I'll just smooth these areas.
8/3 12:00 P.M.	Pick at cuticles	Yes—15 minutes	Nervousness, restless	I'm doing it again. Well, I have to get rid of this loose skin or it will really bother me.

Triggers and Consequences Record

Date and Time	Type of Urge	Emotional Trigger "I felt . . ."	Situational Trigger "I was . . ."	Consequence of Action

Chart 11c

Delia's Triggers and Consequences Record

Date and Time	Type of Urge	Emotional Trigger "I felt . . ."	Situational Trigger "I was . . ."	Consequence of Action
8/2 7:00 A.M.	Pick blemishes on face	Disgusted by look of face. Afraid I wouldn't look right.	Getting ready for work.	Face looked worse after picking at pimples. I tried to cover them up with makeup.
8/2 10:00 A.M.	Pick at cuticles	Nervous about meeting.	Sitting at my desk, thinking about a meeting coming up. I found myself picking, then I needed to fix what I'd picked.	Fingers bleeding and sore. I had to wash and put pressure on my fingers before the meeting.
8/2 3:00 P.M.	Pick at cuticles	Nervous and bored, proud that I didn't pick.	Sitting at my desk and doing paperwork.	Stopped myself before started picking. I felt strong.
8/2 7:00 P.M.	Pick at blemishes on face	Disgusted by look of my face.	Looked in the mirror in the bathroom.	My face was sore and had reddened areas.
8/2 10:00 P.M.	Pick at blemishes on face	Disgusted by what I did to my face, anxious about what I will look like tomorrow.	Getting ready for bed.	Picking didn't help the blemishes look any better and my face was sore.
8/3 8:00 A.M.	Pick at blemishes on face	Worried about looking right today.	Getting ready for work.	I was too embarrassed to face people, so I stayed home from work.
8/3 12:00 P.M.	Pick at cuticles	Anxious about staying home from work. Disgusted that I let the appearance of my face influence my work.	Sitting and watching TV. I felt a rough cuticle.	Fingers looked worse, and I felt discouraged.

Chart 11d

Step 2: List Advantages and Disadvantages

What are the advantages or benefits of keeping your habit? Let's put it another way: What do you get out of this habit? Before you answer, remember that relief from stress and anxiety may be considered a benefit. Picking at her cuticles or face temporarily relieved Delia's anxiety about her appearance; while she was engaged in her habit she would feel that she was doing something to improve her appearance. Afterward, she would see that picking was only making the situation worse. Similarly, wearing loose clothing to cover perceived body-shape defects might actually make a person look less attractive. Often in BDD, the behaviors that are meant to fix blemishes and defects actually do the opposite.

Fill in the boxes in the Advantages and Disadvantages worksheet. Then look at your results. Are the advantages of changing and the disadvantages of keeping your habit more important to you than the reasons not to change? If so, you are ready to change your habit. If not, you may not be ready to give up this habit. Delia found that the advantages of changing far outweighed the advantages of continuing to pick at her skin.

Step 3: Identify Preceding Behaviors

What leads to your habit? Review your Habit Triggers and Consequences chart (above). What emotions and situations usually precede your habit? For people with trichotillomania, a preceding behavior might be running fingers through their hair or twirling their hair. Smoothing his hair with his hand usually preceded Leo's urge to find a mirror and check his hair. Paul's preceding behavior was showing up at the gym and watching his bodybuilder friends work out. Describe exactly what happens just before you engage in your habit. Write your description below.

_____

_____

_____

Delia: *Touching my face and fingers to feel for rough areas, and looking in the mirror, then drawing closer to examine my face are things I do before actually picking.*

_____

_____

Habit Advantages and Disadvantages

Advantages of Keeping the Habit	Disadvantages of Keeping the Habit

Advantages of Changing the Habit	Disadvantages of Changing the Habit

Delia's Habit Advantages and Disadvantages

Advantages of Keeping the Habit	Disadvantages of Keeping the Habit
Relief of anxiety and nervousness. Feeling like I'm fixing my looks.	My face and cuticles will continue to look bad. My face and cuticles don't get a chance to heal. People stare at my face and cuticles. I'm always thinking about the appearance of my skin. Picking makes my skin look worse.

Advantages of Changing the Habit	Disadvantages of Changing the Habit
My face and fingers will probably look better. My face and fingers won't hurt. People won't stare at my face and fingers. I won't look so nervous. I won't be thinking about the appearance of my skin as much. I'll feel stronger, more in control.	The skin around my cuticles and blemishes will be rough while healing. I won't be able to use the habit to relieve anxiety and nervousness.

Chart 11f

Step 4: Identify Habit-Provoking Situations

Now we are going to look at your habit a little differently. Review your Habit Records, your Habit Triggers and Consequences Records, and your answers in step 3. What kind of mood are you usually in when your habit shows up? For example, are you tense, angry, sad, bored, tired, or lonely? Where are you likely to be when you engage in your habit? At what time of day do you seem most vulnerable? Are you usually alone or with someone? Whom are you with? Do you feel more vulnerable while doing certain activities or in particular situations? Answering these questions below will help you identify when you are most likely to engage in your habit. This awareness will help you be on the lookout for habit-provoking situations.

_____

_____

_____

_____

Delia: *I am usually alone in the bathroom and feeling disgusted by my looks when I pick at my face. I can be anywhere and usually feel anxious, nervous, or bored when I pick at my fingers.*

Step 5: Develop a Competing Response

One of the most important steps of habit reversal is to develop a competing response, a behavior you will try to engage in every time you have an urge to start the problem habit. Because you may use it quite frequently, choose a competing response that can be done often and as long as needed. Be sure that the competing response is one you can continue for several minutes. The behavior must be incompatible with your habit. Your competing response should also be a behavior that can be done without interfering with other activities.

Engaging in your competing response should help you become more aware of what you are doing and what you are not doing. While you are engaging in your competing response, continue to remind yourself of the reason you are doing it. This increased awareness of your behavior will help keep you from engaging in your habit without being aware of it.

List several behaviors you could engage in when you are in a habit-provoking situation. Brainstorm—list possible competing responses, without overthinking them. You will eventually choose just one, but for now list at least five from which you can choose.

Possible Competing Responses

1. _____

2. _____

3. _____

4. _____

5. _____

6. _____

7. _____

8. _____

Chart 11g

Delia's Possible Competing Responses

1. _Fold hands in front of me._

2. _Clench a soft ball in each hand._

3. _Play with clay._

4. _Hold a pen in one hand._

5. _Pinch together thumb and forefinger on one or both hands._

6. _Mentally count to 100._

7. _Clench fists._

8. _Work on a jigsaw puzzle._

Chart 11h

After you have listed your possible competing responses, pick one that seems to fit all of the criteria we discussed. It must be a behavior that

- is incompatible with your habit,

- you can do as often as needed,

- you can do as long as the urge continues, and

- can be done without significantly interfering with other activities.

Delia listed eight possible competing responses. After reviewing her list and the criteria above, she eliminated all but one behavior. Clenching a soft ball, playing with clay, holding a pen, or working on a jigsaw puzzle wouldn't work when the items weren't readily available, and doing these things would interfere with other activities. Mentally counting to 100 would not keep her from picking because her hands would still be free. Clenching her fists would make her nervous, she decided. Pinching together her thumb and forefinger, either with her right hand, the one she usually picked with, or with both hands, fit all the criteria. Paul had to get pretty creative with his competing response. He decided to make plans to go somewhere or meet someone immediately after his thirty minutes at the gym. It worked best when the plans involved someone else and he felt obligated to keep an appointment.

From your list, choose the competing response that works best for you. You will be replacing your old habit, with all of its disadvantages and negative consequences, with a new, healthy habit—your competing response. You have already charted the advantages and disadvantages of keeping and changing your habit. Let's do the same with your competing response. Make copies of the Advantages and Disadvantages worksheet. Complete it for the competing response you think will best meet the criteria. If you aren't convinced that this is the best one, complete a chart for another competing response. You may even want to line up more than one competing response, for use in different situations. We've provided Delia's Competing Response Advantages and Disadvantages worksheet as an example.

Like Delia, you may find that the left-hand column of your Competing Response Advantages and Disadvantages worksheet looks much like the left-hand side of your Habit Advantages and Disadvantages worksheet. And, like Delia, you probably won't be able to come up with many disadvantages of your competing response. Delia wrote down her disadvantages, then immediately argued against them. It was clear to her that hers was a good competing response.

When you have found the competing response that works best for you, describe it below. Describe it very specifically this time. Anytime you find yourself engaging in your habit, interrupt it by using your competing response.

_____

_____

_____

_____

Competing Response Advantages and Disadvantages

Competing Response: _____

Advantages	Disadvantages

Delia's Competing Response Advantages and Disadvantages

Competing Response: _Pinching my thumb and forefinger, either one hand or both_

Advantages	Disadvantages
I can't pick and pinch together my finger and thumb at the same time.	I might get tired of this behavior, but if I did, I could try clenching my fists or clutching an object.
Since I usually pick with my right hand, I could pinch either just my right hand or both.	It might not relieve my anxiety and nervousness—then I could practice relaxation.
I could pinch with my right hand and do something else with my left hand, so it doesn't interfere with other activities.	
It wouldn't interfere with most activities.	
People wouldn't notice.	
I would have intact, healthy skin.	
My fingers and face wouldn't hurt so much.	
People wouldn't stare at my fingers and face.	
I would look and feel more in control.	

Chart 11j

Delia: *When I feel the urge to pick at my skin, I will pinch together my thumb and fore-finger, either on one hand or both. I will also do this whenever I find myself touching my face or fingers, feeling for rough spots.*

Step 6: Rehearse Your Competing Response

In step 3 you listed the behaviors that lead up to your engaging in your habit. If you didn't list these behaviors, go back and do so now. Whenever you notice these behaviors, begin your competing response. Rehearse the response now. Think about finding yourself doing one of your preliminary behaviors and stopping yourself. Perform the competing response as you described it in step 5.

Now think about the situations in which you are prone to engage in your habit, which you identified in step 4. If you skipped step 4 because it seemed too obvious and simple, go back and list the situations now. Imagine yourself in one of the habit-provoking situations, performing a few of your preliminary behaviors. Instead of engaging in your habit, start your competing response. Perform your competing response for three to five minutes, and then repeat the exercise three to five times for a total of fifteen minutes.

As you are rehearsing, talk to yourself, either aloud or in your head. Mentally discuss what you are doing, what steps you are taking, and how you are feeling. Most people have anxiety or discomfort associated with the urge or tension that precedes engaging in a habit. It is common to have thoughts such as "I am not going to be able to stand it," "I'm going to go crazy," or "I must do this; I have to do my habit." Talk back to these thoughts, saying, "I haven't gone crazy yet, and sometimes I have resisted my habit," or "The urges will go away. They always do." Chapters 8 and 9 give you more pointers on how to talk back to your negative thoughts.

It is important to rehearse your competing response every day. Plan to dedicate at least fifteen minutes to this each day for seven days. Each day, when you have done your daily rehearsal, check off the days below.

Day 1 _____   Day 2 _____   Day 3 _____   Day 4 _____   Day 5 _____   Day 6 _____   Day 7 _____

By the end of that week the urges will probably have diminished greatly. You may find the habit has almost disappeared. Then you can relax a bit and rehearse only when you feel the urges increasing.

Step 7: Reward Yourself for Your Good Work

Changing habits is hard work. Set small goals for yourself and reward yourself with something special when you've met them. One of Delia's overall goals was to stop picking at blemishes on her face. At first, to go through an entire day without checking her face in the mirror seemed almost impossible. She set an intermediate goal of checking her face for only ten minutes three times a day. When she succeeded, she rewarded herself with a lunch date with a friend, and then she set another goal.

CHAPTER 12

The Role of Self-Esteem

S elf-Esteem is an important topic in dealing with body-image problems. We are going to address the question of self-esteem in this chapter, but we expect that you may want to explore this topic more on your own. For that reason, we've listed some for helpful books on the subject in the Resources section.

Self-Respect and Self-Esteem

My *Webster's New Universal Unabridged Dictionary* (1983) dictionary defines self-esteem as "belief in oneself; self-respect." Closely related is the idea of *self-concept,* which might be defined as what you think of yourself or your ideas about yourself. The difference is that self-esteem has to do with value. If we hold something in esteem, we believe it has some value or worth. Your self-concept includes facts such as your age, marital status, job, name, and other information about you. It may also include ideas about qualities or traits you believe you have; you may think of yourself as smart or dumb, a good athlete or a klutz, a hard worker or a lazy bum, good looking or ugly.

As we said above, some elements of self-concept are based on fact: "I have brown eyes; I have dark hair; I am married." Other elements are based on our opinions: "I am good looking; I am a kind person; I am smart." Other elements are based on speculation about what others think: "People know I am thoughtful and hardworking; my friends think I am smart; people think I am ugly." Many of these elements may fall somewhere on a continuum. With other elements, you may see yourself as being at the extreme end of the continuum, or you may view your appearance in an all-or-nothing way: "I am good looking" or "I am ugly," with no in-between. If you happen to think in an all-or-nothing way about your appearance, and you are reading this book because of your own body-image dissatisfaction, it is likely that you put yourself in the ugly group. You may want to go back and look at the discussion of absolute thinking in chapters 8 and 9.

Self-esteem is based on the value or importance we assign to the components of our self-concept. In other words, if your self-concept includes beliefs like "I am pretty smart, I am a moral person, and I have a very ugly nose," and you think the first two are important and the third is not important, you are likely to have reasonably good self-esteem. Think of this as an algebraic equation. All of the different parts of self-concept add up to make the total. Of course, you may think of something as subtracting rather than adding.

Look back at the example above of the person who sees himself or herself as smart and moral, but as having an ugly nose. The person still has reasonably good self-esteem because the positive features add up and the negative one, the ugly nose, does not subtract much. Cameron, however, put a lot of value on having an attractive nose. For him, the formula was changed; most of his positive traits were unimportant to him, and the negative element of self-concept, the ugly nose, was the only one with any real importance. That made it quite likely that he would have a serious problem with low self-esteem. If you have body-image dissatisfaction, you will probably find that you have low self-esteem. You give a lot of importance to parts of your self-concept that are related to your appearance, and you think of those elements of your self-concept in very negative or all-or-noth4 ing terms. But you aren't alone; many people are struggling with just this kind of problem.

Examine Your Self-Concept

Let's look at the elements of your self-concept, then try to understand how they add up to your self-esteem. Make copies of the Self-Concept Exploration worksheet, which follows, and fill it out. List as many descriptions of yourself as you can think of. Then identify whether each item is based on fact (F), your opinion (O), or what you believe others think (OT). Finally, assign each item an importance rating, according to how important you hold this part of your self-concept to be (0 being least important, and 10 being most important). Indicate whether this item is positive (P) and adds to your total self-esteem, or negative (N) and subtracts from your self-esteem. Work on this worksheet each day for a week. You may need several copies in order to list all of your descriptions of yourself. We've provided Cameron's form as an example.

As you look at the self-concepts and evaluations that make up your self-esteem, you will probably find that they seem to fit into a small number of categories, accomplishments, appearance traits, personality traits, and others' opinions of you. For example, Cherry thought that the *accomplishments* of doing well in school and getting a good job were reasons for positive self-esteem. On the other hand, you may have noted that some aspect of your *appearance* was a reason for negative self-esteem. Cameron had very low self-esteem because of one appearance trait.

The *opinions of others* can be a powerful influence on self-esteem and can modify the importance of any of the other categories. For example, if Cherry thought it was important to have done well in school, not so much because it meant something to her, but because it meant other people would look up to her, then other people's opinions would really be a key to her self-esteem. The same could be true of appearance or personality traits. Often, some combination of the importance of the accomplishment or trait and the beliefs about other's opinions that make up a person's overall self-esteem.

All these sources of self-esteem come with some problems. What if you derived your self-esteem from accomplishments? There is the risk of basing your self-esteem on what you have accomplished *lately*. Even if you have made it to the top of your field or are the best in your group, what happens when you slip? Even the best athlete will lose some games, or get older and no longer be able to do things he or she once could. A similar problem is associated with appearance. Even the most beautiful people lose some of their good looks with age. What happens if you get a scar or gain weight, or get older? Even basing self-esteem on personality traits is risky. One problem is that we often think about these traits in absolute terms. If I think I am an honest person and then I do some minor dishonest things, I may start thinking that I am not an honest person, and there goes my self-esteem.

Even those traits we see in relative terms can be a problem. If I think I am a smart person and meet someone who is clearly much smarter, I may start to feel bad. When we tie our self-esteem to someone else's opinion, we have to guess what they think in the first place. We also have to guess what they are paying attention to and the importance they give to us and our traits. For example, Cameron thinks everyone looks at his nose, thinks it's ugly, and doesn't want him around. How does he know that *anyone* is looking at his nose, much less *everyone*? How does he know that anyone is thinking it is ugly or that people don't want him around because of it? They may or may not want Cameron around, but it may or may not be connected to his nose.

Self Concept Exploration

Item	Description	Basis	Importance

Chart 12a

Cameron's Self Concept Exploration

Item	Description	Basis	Importance
1	I have brown eyes.	F	1 P
2	I am a hard worker.	O	4 P
3	I have a big and very ugly nose.	O, OT	9 N
4	I dropped out of high school.	F	4 N
5	Because of number 4 everyone knows I am stupid.	OT	6 N
6	I am an honest person.	O, OT	4 P
7	I am tall.	F	2 P
8	I have been told that I have a nice smile.	OT	3 P
9	I get angry sometimes.	F	5 N
10	I get anxious easily.	O	5 N
11	I am dependable.	O, OT	4 P
12	My hair is brown.	F	2 P
13	My hair is naturally curly and unruly.	O	3 N
14	People say that I am moody.	OT	4 N
15	I help people when I see that they need it.	O, OT	4 P
16	I am overweight, according to the charts.	F	3 N
17	I have a mustache.	F	2 P
18	I have relatively dry skin.	F	1 N
19	I worry a lot about what other people think.	F	7 N
20	I think too much about the way my nose looks.	O	8 N

Why Do We Care What Other People Think?

Let's think a little about why we place such great importance on the opinions of others. If you believe that other people's evaluations of you or your appearance are important, there has to be some reason for this belief. Some people say they want people to like them. That sounds reasonable, but it wouldn't be hard to find someone who didn't like you. For example, if you are an American, it would be easy to find people in other parts of the world who hate you because of your nationality. You might respond that you're not bothered by that since you don't like them either, or that their dislike of you is just the result of prejudice.

If you can dismiss some people's opinions that easily, what thinking underlies your belief that the opinions of others are so important? You might say, "I want people who know me to like me." If you believe they won't like you because of one of your traits or accomplishments, ask yourself, "Do I think that way?" Do you dislike people who have not accomplished much? Do you dislike people who are not perfect in their appearance? Would you not want to be friends with someone because he had a scar or an ugly nose? You probably think that that is ridiculous—perhaps you find pretty people more attractive, but you don't think of them as better or more worthwhile.

Similarly, you may admire someone who seems to have accomplished a great deal or who has admirable personality traits, but this doesn't mean that you like that person. For example, you might consider someone who has risen to the office of president of the United States to have accomplished a great deal, but you may not agree with him on important issues, or you may think he is unlikable, uncaring.

Realistically, most of the people in the world don't know you exist. Of those who do, some may like you, some may not, and some may not have much of an opinion either way. Even those who do know you are not likely to spend a lot of time thinking about you. Even if we suppose that the few people who think about you do think only positive things, does that make you a better person? What if their opinions are mixed? Consider the president again. Some people may think he is a great man. Others are likely to think some very negative things about him. If his worth is dependent on their opinions, does it go up and down with the opinion polls?

Self-Esteem and Value

You may be asking yourself what else can be used to help determine self-esteem. We seem to have discarded all the usual factors you might use. This is a question many philosophers have tried to answer, with various degrees of success. If we can't determine self-esteem using our accomplishments, appearance, personality traits, or even what others think, what is left? There are a few different answers to this question, two of which are presented below.

One answer is that every human has some intrinsic worth. Some people may find this expressed in their religious faith. The Quakers teach, "There is that of God in everyone." This can be understood as saying that we all have some goodness or value that can't be taken away. It could be understood simply that human life has value. The value is not something that can be measured. It is not something that is increased by accomplishment or the approval of others. It is not decreased by failure or disapproval. If this idea is one that is comfortable for you, then next time you use traits and accomplishments to determine your self-worth, stop and remind yourself that those things don't really add up after all. You simply need to understand that you are worthwhile.

Another answer is that our worth is not something we can meaningfully determine. Using this belief, we can learn to simply accept that the pursuit of some measure of self-esteem is a futile exercise and stop trying to figure out where we fit on the imaginary scale. If you base your self-esteem, your value as a human being, on your works or appearance or the opinions of others, can you ever measure up? There will always be someone who can perform better or who is more attractive. That would mean that we are all worthless at times and worthwhile at times. But how can we be both? Could it be that worthlessness just doesn't exist? If you measure yourself using one set of criteria, you would be worthwhile; using another you would be worthless.

Some might argue that we are all flawed—that we were born flawed. Any deviation from perfection could be considered a flaw. If we were not flawed, we would all be the same and we would all be perfect. But are we really flawed, or just different? Does perfection even exist? Let's assume for a moment that we are flawed. That would mean that we have room for improvement, and that could give us purpose, problems to overcome, and goals to achieve. If we were perfect, what purpose would we have? Perhaps it is good that we aren't perfect or unflawed—it gives us a purpose.

Mindfulness and Value

The study of mindfulness can help us with this concept. If we accept either of the above answers about self-esteem we can also accept that we are what we are and that we do not need to judge ourselves. Part of mindfulness is to observe without judging. Methods of judging our self-worth or measuring self-esteem by adding up accomplishments, appearance traits , personality traits, or opinions of others all involve judgments. These can be our own judgments or those we suspect others have made. It is ironic that most of us would say being judgmental is not a trait we want to have, and that we would not admire it in others, but we apply it unhesitatingly to ourselves.

Too often we label ourselves using only a few characteristics or roles, and many of us place more importance on the negative traits. What if we mindfully consider the other categories we fit into? Don't mindlessly accept labels. When we label ourselves or others, we focus on one particular characteristic. But when we take a closer look, we discover that even a severe disability can help a person in other areas. A blind person can mindfully attend to other senses. A person who has experienced anxiety can have greater empathy for others who are anxious or frightened.

When we label ourselves and others we look at the world in a black or white fashion. People are ugly or beautiful, short or tall, thin or fat. But when we get rid of the labels, we can find unlimited variations within categories. The labels *worthwhile* and *worthless* become less meaningful or become a question without an answer. We can be described as having more or less of some traits, but we are not labeled in absolute terms.

 Image Balancing Strategy

Labels are useful for identifying varieties of soup, but they aren't effective ways of describing people. Stay away from labeling yourself and others.

Self-Critical Thoughts

As you've learned throughout this book, changing how you think changes how you feel. As you change your thoughts about yourself, your feelings will also change, resulting in a comfortable self-image and sense of self-esteem. Review your Self-Image Journal, and on a separate sheet of paper create a list of thoughts that are self-critical, using the distorted thoughts you wrote on your Alternative Body-Image Thoughts worksheets (chapter 8). In your daily life look for negative comparisons you make between yourself and others, and any inflated importance you give to negative characteristics, other people's opinions, and your control of characteristics and circumstances, and add these self-critical thoughts to your list. Then list more realistic alternative thoughts. For example, you might have the thought, "I have a big, ugly nose." An alternative might be "I have a large nose." It contains the same idea about size, but not the judgment that it is ugly. If the criticism is from others who say you have a big, ugly nose, you could think, "It is true, I have a larger-than-average nose and some people might think it is ugly, but that is simply their opinion, not a fact." You may even want to write the alternatives on separate three-by-five-inch cards. Review these when you find yourself thinking self-critical thoughts. These alternative thoughts aren't merely affirmations that may or may not be true. They are positive, realistic, honest statements. We tend to believe negative thoughts about ourselves, but we aren't likely to believe positive thoughts. Teach yourself to believe your alternative thoughts, reviewing them as often as necessary.

 Image Balancing Strategy

Replace self-critical distorted thoughts with positive, realistic, honest statements. Review them daily, adding more as you find them.

Criticism from others can be handled the same way. List the criticisms on a blank Alternative Body-Image Thoughts chart, and then list more realistic statements on a separate sheet of paper. What can you learn from the criticisms? You may find that there is no evidence to support the statements. Statements without support can simply be dismissed.

But what if there is some evidence to support the critical statements from others or from yourself? What do you do if, after you've restated them in a more realistic way, they're still negative? Work toward accepting and even embracing these characteristics. When you accept that you, like every human being, are not perfect, the negative impact is muted. You still have the flaw, but it doesn't matter as much since it is evidence that you are human. If it still seems important, you can decide, without the interference of emotions, whether change is necessary.

A mindful response to your negative thoughts about your accomplishments, your appearance, your personality traits, or the opinions of others might include noticing they exist, observing and experiencing the thoughts, and allowing them to be part of your human experience without giving them weight or importance—in other words, without judgment. If you look back at chapters 8 and 9, you will recognize that the distortions in thinking that contribute to problems with self-esteem, depression, and anxiety are really all forms of judgment. Being mindful is a way of stopping the self-criticism and self-abuse that contributes to negative self-esteem.

Finally, let's consider treating ourselves like we would a valued friend. If you would treat a valued friend with respect, then do so for yourself. If you would never judge your friends harshly because they had not accomplished as much as they could have or because they aren't attractive, treat yourself the same way. If you would truly love or accept others even if they were horribly deformed or ugly, then treat yourself the same way.

CHAPTER 13

Social Isolation

People with BDD or serious body-image dissatisfaction are almost always overly concerned about what others are going to think of their appearance or how others are going to react to them. Naturally, if you think some part of your body is distorted and ugly, you will expect others to think the same, and surely if others see this defect or ugliness they will be distressed by it, want to avoid it, or think negative things about you. Consider Jamila, who thought her fingers were much too long and her hands were disgustingly large. Whenever she went out in public, she had obsessive thoughts about other people looking at her hands and being offended. Since she thought that what others were thinking was very important and truly believed that almost everyone who saw her had such thoughts, she found going out extremely uncomfortable and painful.

It's the most natural thing in the world to try to stop anxiety and distress by getting out of stressful situations and avoiding experiences that have been painful in the past. In fact, it is important for our survival to learn from painful experiences. Our brains are built to learn these lessons quickly and change our behavior to avoid pain in the future. Although in this case the pain is emotional, the learning process is the same. This kind of learning is at the core of social avoidance in people with body-image problems. In order to overcome it, you are going to have to do some very hard work.

Help and Hope for Social Anxiety Disorder

This book is about BDD and related body-image problems, but let's talk briefly about a social problem that often results from BDD. People who spend a lot of time avoiding social contact and have significant anxiety whenever they are in social situations may also fit the diagnostic criteria for one of the most common disorders in mental health. *Social anxiety disorder* (also called social phobia) is characterized by a marked and persistent fear of social and/or performance situations, with concern about negative evaluations by others or embarrassment. Some researchers have estimated that as many as 13 percent of the population could be diagnosed with social anxiety disorder. This means that perhaps thirteen people out of every one hundred have enough social anxiety that it causes them significant distress and interferes with their lives. Many more have some social anxiety in specific situations such as public speaking or performing. Most of the people in this latter group probably simply manage to avoid most of the situations where they would be called on to perform.

A second diagnosis may also apply; some experts believe that *avoidant personality disorder* is best understood as a more severe form of social anxiety disorder, with which it overlaps. It is characterized by a pervasive pattern of social isolation, inhibition, and feelings of inadequacy, with hypersensitivity to criticism, disapproval, or negative evaluations by others. People with this disorder can spend their whole lives in isolation and fear. How common are avoidant personality disorder and social anxiety disorder in people with BDD? Katharine Phillips (1996) reports that 26 percent of people with BDD will meet the criteria for social phobia at any given time and 36 percent will meet the criteria for social phobia at some point in their life. Phillips and Susan McElroy (2000) found that 43 percent of people with BDD met the criteria for avoidant personality disorder in their sample.

These numbers demonstrate that a large percentage of people with BDD have enough social impairment to meet criteria for a second disorder. It is reasonable to expect that almost everyone with BDD, and many people with less severe body-image problems, have some degree of social anxiety and as a result restrict their social interactions or withdraw from others. Phillips (1996) has also suggested that BDD may be missed in a significant number of people who are diagnosed with social anxiety disorder, often because clinicians simply don't ask the right questions. We would speculate that this is also true for people diagnosed with avoidant personality disorder. These theories correspond with the finding that a large number of people treated for depression have unrecognized BDD (Phillips 1996). We can conclude that most people who have serious body-image problems also have some social anxiety problems.

You may be thinking, "Oh, great, now I have something else wrong with me." Well, you may or you may not. Even if you don't have diagnosable social anxiety disorder, you very likely have enough anxiety in social situations to be able to benefit from the same treatment principles used for the disorder. The good news is that we know a lot about treating social anxiety problems, and we know that the treatment works well. The best treatment for social anxiety is cognitive behavioral therapy. Many of the things you have learned already are really parts of the set of tools you will need to deal with social anxiety. Answer these questions about yourself to see if your body-image problem is causing some problems in connecting to others socially.

1. Do you avoid going to public places because of concerns about your appearance?

2. Do you refuse social invitations because of concerns about your appearance?

3. Do you avoid dating or other romantic interpersonal relationships because of concerns about your appearance or expectation of rejection related to appearance?

4. Do you avoid eye contact, standing close to other people, or personal contact such as shaking hands or hugging because of concerns about your appearance?

5. Do you avoid sexual activity or being seen by a sexual partner because of concerns about your appearance?

If you answered "yes" to any of these questions, your body-image concern is causing problems in your social interactions. If social anxiety is a significant problem for you, then in addition to doing the exercises here you may want to check out the information we've included in the Resources section.

Examine the Evidence for Negative Social Events

Looking back at your work in chapters 8 and 9, you'll notice that many of your distorted thoughts involve social situations. Replacing these with alternative thoughts that are more realistic will help you put your fears into perspective. If you didn't address distorted thoughts about social situations in those chapters, go back and do so now. Look for thoughts that overestimate the probability of the occurrence of embarrassing or painful social situations. Look also for thoughts that overestimate the severity of potentially negative social situations. Would the consequences really be as severe as you fear? Usually not.

Now, we are going to teach you to approach your life like a scientist. This means coming up with a hypothesis about what will happen in a situation, and then testing it by collecting evidence. Let's consider Jamila. She answered "yes" to questions 1 through 4 above. She didn't have a partner at this point, so question 5 didn't apply.

After Jamila wrote her hypothesis, Dr. Claiborn tried to help her see that perhaps her hypothesis was unrealistic. So she came up with an alternative hypothesis. She didn't really believe it, but she agreed to humor Dr. Claiborn and test her original hypothesis. Jamila began to list the evidence that would prove her original hypothesis. But Jamila was not proving to be a very good scientist. She viewed any event as evidence to confirm her original hypothesis. If people looked at her, it meant they were disgusted with her looks; if they didn't look at her, they were disgusted. She couldn't win! She needed to define, more specifically, what would qualify as evidence that others found her hands disgusting. After much consideration, she listed more realistic evidence that would support her belief. Now it was time to do the experiment. Jamila agreed to go to the mall (at a time when it was not too crowded, so it would be less anxiety-producing) and make some observations. Then she came to the most critical step: the interpretation of her findings. How did Jamila interpret the observations? Does the data support her hypothesis or does it support the alternative one?

Hypothesis: *If I go out in public everyone will stare at my hands and see how long my fingers are. They will be repulsed and disgusted.*

Alternative hypothesis: *If I go out in public people will not react to me any differently than they do to anyone else.*

Expected evidence: *People either stare at my hands, or they don't look at me at all because they see how disgusting I look and then look away.*

Concrete evidence: *Small children point at my hands and ask their parents what is wrong with me. A clerk in a store says, "Your hands are huge!" Strangers gasp as I pass them and examine their hands to make sure they haven't suddenly become distorted like mine.*

Observations: *None of the things I listed as concrete evidence occurred. I "felt" people staring at me, but when I checked most people seemed to simply glance at me and then look away. My heart was beating very fast, and I felt very uncomfortable, but the clerk in the store was polite and seemed willing to wait on me.*

Interpretation: *People's reaction to me at the mall did not support my original hypothesis. People seemed to react to me as if I was normal looking. Even though I was very uncomfortable, nothing really bad seemed to happen.*

It's time for you to set up an experiment to test your social anxiety concerns. Follow the model we have laid out and fill in the blanks below. Begin with a testable hypothesis. It has to be one that can be checked out by gathering data. That means it can't be an opinion. "I'm ugly" is an opinion. "Because I am ugly people will not look at me" is a testable idea. You don't have to believe your alternative hypothesis yet; you only need to accept it as an idea you are willing to try out. Remember that you are setting out to be a scientist. Look at your expected evidence. Are you making the mistake of assuming what you are trying to prove? Is *any* outcome going to prove what you already believe? Try to come up with what others would accept as concrete evidence. The toughest part of your experiment will be testing your hypothesis by going into a situation you usually avoid and making observations about what actually happens. Finally, evaluate the evidence and decide which hypothesis it supports.

Hypothesis: _____

_____

Alternative hypothesis: _____

_____

Expected evidence: _____

_____

Concrete evidence: _____

_____

_____

_____

Observations: _____

_____

_____

_____

Interpretation: _____

_____

_____

Any scientist will tell you that real science involves repeatable experiments. You'll need to repeat your experiment a number of times. Each time, review the evidence and see which hypothesis it supports. You may want to start out with situations that are not too upsetting or frightening. As you do the experiments, you can also keep track of how uncomfortable you are in the situation and see if that changes over time. When one sort of situation gets easier to deal with, you can move on to a more difficult one.

Image Balancing Strategy

Use imaginal exposure and response change to gain strength and confidence for upcoming social situations.

Behavioral Change

The information in chapter 7 can also help you feel more comfortable in social situations. Continue to practice daily relaxation exercises at home. By now, you can probably become relaxed within a few minutes. Use your skills to obtain a relaxed state when you first enter a social situation, and at regular intervals while you are in the situation.

The exposure exercises in chapter 10 will also be helpful. Add social situations to your hierarchy of stressful situations. Working on these situations will require some creativity. After all, you can't always give a speech or attend a party often enough to bring down your anxiety level. This is where a special type of exposure works well. We taught you *in vivo* (real-life) exposures in chapter 10. With social situations, you can start with *imaginal* exposure.

Sit comfortably and use one of your relaxation techniques from chapter 7 for a few minutes. Now, take one of the low-level or mid-level situations from your hierarchy and imagine it actually happening. Weave a story in your mind, including details of what could occur. The events may be based on what has happened in the past or on what you fear could happen. Allow your anxiety to rise and peak as you experience the embarrassment, fear, and distress. If the anxiety becomes too severe, use your relaxation skills only until it becomes bearable, then go back to your imaginary situation. Don't stop, though. Since this is imaginary, you can soften the situation a bit, but it is important to follow yourself through the entire situation. If you're imagining giving a speech, finish the speech and sit down. If you're imagining going to a party, see yourself home.

Continue with your imaginal exposures daily. When you feel little or no anxiety in one imagined situation, go on to another. You may find it easier to record your story on a tape recorder and play it repeatedly. Or try writing it out as a script and reading it to yourself repeatedly. The important thing is to experience the anxiety and learn that it is tolerable. Even if the things you fear come to pass, you can handle them. When you've successfully dealt with a social situation in your mind, go on to an *in vivo* situation. Imaginal exposure is a good way to prepare yourself for feared social situations. Use it daily for several days before a speech, party, date, or even encounters with coworkers, acquaintances, or friends. Don't forget the unexpected, the dreaded, such as dropping all your notes during a speech or spilling food or drink at a dinner. You can handle anything.

Mindfulness and Mindlessness in Social Situations

People with social anxiety often engage in some behaviors that perpetuate the problem. When in social situations you may be paying attention to cues from your own body and thoughts and using them to predict what others are thinking, how well you are fitting in, or whether you are being rejected. It is common to notice you are feeling uncomfortable and assume that this means you are making others uncomfortable. You may avoid eye contact, then notice that others are not talking to you, and assume this means that you are not accepted, when in fact others are reading your avoidance of eye contact as a signal that you don't want to talk. Or you may obsess about the appearance of a body part and, since you can't stop thinking about it, assume that others are equally focused on it.

This internal or self-focused attention may also lead you to miss many of the cues in social interactions. Someone who is interested in talking to you may try to make eye contact. However, if you are busy looking at your shoes, you can't tell. Many people with BDD or other body-image concerns worry about features of their face. If you see someone looking at your face, you may assume that the person is looking at the "problem" feature.

This is where you can use what we've learned about mindfulness. You can decide what to be mindful about and what to be "mindless" about. Rarely is focusing on a performance *during* the performance helpful—during a performance of any type, it is best not to judge your performance. By being mindful, you will be less focused on judging your performance or your appearance. Be mindful of your surroundings, your experiences, and your thoughts by observing them, not reacting to them. It can even be valuable to mindfully observe what others are doing.

We are coming to the end of the Balanced Image Program. You are likely feeling less anxiety about and dissatisfaction with your appearance, but you probably aren't "cured." Your healing will likely be a lifelong endeavor. The next chapter will help you maintain the gains you've made and continue your efforts to achieve a balanced body image.

CHAPTER 14

Maintaining Your Gains

By this time you are probably well into the action stage of change and entering the maintenance stage. Many people think this is the end of the process of change, that they've made it. Don't make this mistake. Maintenance is every bit as important as action. This chapter will help you make your changes permanent.

Relapse Prevention

When researchers looked at the outcome of the treatments of substance abuse, it became clear that they needed to come up with some new ideas. A high percentage of people were not able to maintain the gains that they made in treatment. In other words, relapse rates were disturbingly high. Perhaps you have made efforts to change your body-image-related behaviors or your self-image in the past. You may have started out well, then slipped back gradually or suddenly to your old way of doing things—you relapsed.

One researcher working on alcohol treatment came up with a concept he called *relapse prevention*. Dr. G. A. Marlatt (1985) examined what went wrong in the treatment of people with alcohol problems. How did relapse occur? He developed a set of ideas about what could be done differently and what could be added to treatment that would improve the disturbing relapse rate. These ideas are now used in working with a broad range of behavioral problems. We will discuss these ideas in this chapter, along with some recommendations on relapse and relapse prevention for people with body-image problems.

Does it scare you to think about relapse? It is a common fear. Many people, even well-meaning professionals, think it is a bad idea to talk about relapse. They believe it is important to keep a positive attitude, that even considering relapse could make it more likely to happen. While having a positive attitude is important, dismissing the possibility of relapse can actually make you even more likely to relapse. This is in part because people tend to think in all-or-nothing terms. They think things like, "Either I have a problem or I don't." You may think that either you look good or you look horrible. We don't expect you to get to the point where you never have a thought or worry about how you look. If you expect to get to that point and worries do occur, you may think you have failed and are now back at the starting point. We believe it is better to accept the possibility, or indeed the probability, of the return of some symptoms and prepare for it.

We've discussed the problem of making predictions without evidence. The idea that discussing a problem can make it more likely to occur is that very type of thinking distortion. A more realistic approach is to look at how people successfully maintain changes and what makes them likely to relapse. Accepting the possibility of relapse and understanding its risks will help you plan ways to deal with it.

What Is a Relapse?

Before we discuss how to prevent relapse, we need to be clear about what a relapse is. You've probably heard the word used to describe any return to old habits. We've heard people describe a onetime event as a relapse. A recovering-alcoholic friend of Cherry's referred to one night she spent drinking as a "relapse." This is not a relapse. We use the word to mean a return to your old *pattern* of behavior, or going back to where you were before you started working on your problem. A more appropriate word for a brief episode of the problem behavior is a *lapse*. Cherry's friend had a lapse. If she had continued to drink, the episode would have been termed a relapse. For people with body-image problems or BDD, a lapse may involve going back to compulsively checking in the mirror, avoiding people and places, or picking at skin. It can also include returning to a behavior or way of thinking that was a significant part of their problem.

Maintaining Balance

Why do we make a point of distinguishing between lapses and relapses? Because the difference is critical in spotting the distortions in thinking that are part of the problem. We discussed thinking in absolutes in chapter 9. Also known as an *abstinence violation effect* (AVE), this thinking error can turn a lapse into a relapse. When people try to change a behavior they often think about it in absolute terms: "I used to act that way, but not anymore. I've changed." If they have a lapse, they may switch and start telling themselves that the unwanted behavior is back: "I changed for a while, but then I went back to my old ways." They think of the behavior as uncontrollable, or they think of themselves as powerless over the behavior.

"I've been this way for years. I can't change." How many times have you made this absolute statement? This type of thinking is part of the AVE. Thinking of yourself as powerless, and thinking of yourself as defined by your problems are both forms of absolute thinking, and sources of trouble. How can we avoid the AVE? First, be prepared for lapses, expect them, and be prepared to use the skills you've learned to get back to a balanced body image when they do occur.

Challenge Thoughts and Beliefs about Your Lapse

When the lapse comes, examine your thinking about the lapse. Investigate the thoughts and beliefs that are making you so distressed about the lapse. This will help you stop thinking in absolutes and help you maintain your balance. Complete a Distorted Thought Record whenever a lapse occurs, then choose one of your automatic thoughts and use a flowchart to discover a harmful belief behind it. Create flowcharts for several automatic thoughts until you find the harmful belief that seems to be causing the most trouble, then complete a Problem Belief Challenge worksheet. Each day during the next week, list the evidence you gather that supports the basic belief and evidence that supports the alternative belief.

Deal with High-Risk Situations

High-risk situations are unique to each individual. For some people, high-risk situation might be a stressful day. Stressful times are usually high-risk situations for most people, and it is a good idea to keep this in mind. High-risk situations can be ordinary events, such as walking past a mirror for people with skin picking or hair pulling problems, or they can be unique, unexpected moments. You've probably already run across some high-risk situations for you. Think of other situations you might encounter and list them below.

High-risk situations:

1. _____

2. _____

3. _____

4. _____

High-risk situations can get you heading toward relapse. Handling them appropriately will help you maintain balance. High-risk situations are dangerous because of the automatic thoughts that may occur. In chapters 8 and 9, we discussed the effects of facilitating thoughts. Unfortunately, they may still be around long after you have made significant changes. Write down some of the facilitating thoughts you might have when you get into the high-risk situations you listed above. For each facilitating thought, develop a more reasonable thought. Print them on three-by-five-inch cards and place them where you'll be likely to run into high-risk situations.

The important thing to remember in relapse prevention is that lapses are quite common and likely to occur. You will be better able to handle such problems if you plan ahead. Identify high-risk situations and plan how to deal with them. Learn what sorts of thoughts and beliefs make them a problem. Be especially attentive to absolute statements you make about your character and strength. For example, telling yourself that a lapse means you are a failure will make the lapse more likely to become a relapse. If on the other hand, you tell yourself that this is actually a common problem and that it is simply teaching you something new so you will be better able to handle a high-risk situation in the future, then the lapse will be a valuable learning experience.

 Image Balancing Strategy

Lapses happen. Plan ahead and be prepared to use the skills you've learned here when you encounter high-risk situations. When lapses occur, regroup and get back on track.

Regroup

When a lapse has occurred, go back to the tools that helped before. Examine each part of your work in the Balanced Image Program for weak links. We've already reviewed thinking habits and high-risk situations. What about the rest of the program? Review previous chapters and, below, check off the areas that you need to give more attention.

☐ **Exposure and Response Prevention**
Are your exposure situations challenging enough? Too challenging? Have you stopped doing exposures and retreated to avoidance of certain situations? Review chapter 10 and be creative as you develop more exposure and response-change opportunities.

☐ **Relaxation**
Are you practicing your relaxation exercise daily? If it's not working for you, try one of the other relaxation exercises. If you are not practicing mindful meditation, give that a try. The Resources section lists books that can help you find a better relaxation method for you.

☐ **Record keeping**
Are you still keeping Habit Records of your body-image-related behaviors (chapter 11)? When you begin a lapse, it is especially important to keep records of your problem behaviors so you can clearly see when and how much you are engaging in them.

☐ **Advantages and disadvantages**
The further you get from your body-image-related behaviors and thoughts, the easier it is to forget the disadvantages of the behaviors and thoughts. Review the advantages and disadvantages you recorded in chapter 11. Remind yourself of what life with your unbalanced body image was really like.

☐ **Competing response**
Are your competing responses working? Do they make engaging in your body image related habits impossible? Sometimes we develop ways of doing the competing responses and participating in our habits at the same time. You may need to choose other competing responses, ones that really do interfere with your habits.

☐ **Social support**
Do you have a support person? Does your support person know what type of support you need? Discuss your needs openly and honestly. Read chapter 15 for ideas about how your support person can help. Consider joining a support group or forming your own group.

Achieving a balanced self-image is a challenge. For some people it is a minor change that requires some effort for a short while. For others, the change will be a lifelong endeavor—a very worthwhile endeavor, rich with rewards. Continue the course, and when you find yourself straying, regroup again, and review the Balanced Image Program.

CHAPTER 15

Family Support

The support of family members and significant others is important to the individual who has BDD or serious body-image concerns. You need your family's support as you make changes that lead to a more balanced body image. But wait a minute—let's use what we've learned about examining our automatic thoughts here. Do we really *need* support? What if your family doesn't choose to give you adequate support? So *need* probably isn't the best word. We *want* support. Making a change is usually easier when done with the support of family and friends. If your family can't or won't provide the support, seek it from friends or a support group.

Throughout *The BDD Workbook*, we have instructed you to do things that are leading you toward recovery, including writing down your thoughts and behaviors, doing behavioral experiments, and practicing relaxation. Now you have one last task: show this chapter to someone you care about. Ask that person to read it, and then when they have, sit down and talk it over. With that in mind, we address this chapter to family members and loved ones and hope it will lead to healthy, helpful, open conversations.

Understanding BDD

We all have concerns about particular parts of our bodies that we dislike or find less than ideal. If your family member or friend with BDD expresses dissatisfaction with a body part, you may be inclined to respond, "Yeah, I don't like my nose that much either, but it's no big deal." You may wonder, If I can dismiss the thought and not let it bug me, why can't they just get over it and stop focusing on it?

You may have given reassurance that he or she looked fine many times. Unfortunately, the typical result of this reassurance is that the person with BDD only feels better for a short time. This is a frustrating situation for everyone involved. You probably wish you could say the right thing to make your loved one feel better about their body image. If only you could find the right words to explain that their looks are not distorted the way they think, if only they could feel okay about their appearance, there would be no problem. In addition, people with BDD do other things that seem even more senseless. They may pick at their skin, spend hours trying to fix something that doesn't need fixing, or avoid situations that could actually help them feel better about themselves. It may seem to you that if your loved one could stop these types of behaviors the problem would take care of itself.

The most important thing you can offer is understanding. When your friend or relative tells you that some part of their appearance is a problem, don't dismiss it as vanity or, worse, foolishness. Remember that we are talking about a fundamental part of how they see themselves. Reflect for a moment on how you would feel if you believed you had some personality or appearance trait that made you disgusting or horrible to all who knew you. People with BDD struggle with just this kind of belief. If you have not yet read the first part of this book, you will want to take the time to do so now; it will help you understand this disorder, how common it is, and how agonizing it can be, so you can provide the kind of support your loved one needs.

You can communicate your understanding by listening empathetically. When the person with BDD says, "My _____ looks horrible; I can't go out today," you can respond by saying, "I understand you are upset because you feel like your _____ looks horrible and you don't want to go out. It sounds like you are feeling both disgusted with yourself and afraid." This expresses empathy, but not agreement or reassurance. Below are a few dos and don'ts to keep in mind when dealing with someone with BDD.

- Do express empathy.
- Don't dismiss or invalidate their concerns.
- Do reflectively listen to their concerns.
- Don't give automatic reassurances that everything is fine.
- Do encourage facing the fear.
- Don't criticize them for avoiding frightening situations.
- Do recognize their distress.
- Don't say, "I know just how you feel."

Teasing

Almost everyone has been teased about something. It is a virtually universal experience in childhood and is not uncommon among adults. Most people manage to dismiss teasing or feel only mildly upset about it. Like most people, the majority of those with BDD report some teasing about their appearance in the past. Although it seems unlikely that this is a major reason why some people develop BDD, it certainly feeds the problem. In people with a predisposition to BDD, teasing may serve to focus their body-image concerns and validate the idea that others see it as a problem.

Even among people without BDD, teasing can be hurtful. Sometimes people will tease an adult about some aspect of their appearance and think it is all in good fun. However, the person on the receiving end of the teasing may be hurt but unwilling to speak up about it. Even more hurtful is an attempt to use teasing to try to encourage a person to get over the concern. This approach is almost guaranteed to backfire. Although adults may have some ability to distance themselves from this kind of thing, it is still likely to be damaging. Children are even more vulnerable since they often cannot fully distinguish between teasing and intended messages.

Mindfulness

The concept of mindfulness (see chapter 2) can be useful in your efforts to be supportive. We suggest that you can be most helpful to people with BDD by being mindful when you listen and respond to them. This involves observing but not judging. Observe that they are distressed, that they have a concern about their appearance that is central to their image of themselves, and that this concern is interfering with their lives. Avoid judging the concern as minimal, unimportant, trivial, or wrong. Accept that the problem is real and important to them. Finally, think about how your responses are likely to be received before you utter them.

Now, go to your family member or friend who has BDD and say, "I just read this and I want to talk about it." Ask how you can be supportive. Perhaps you could discuss the exercises as they work on them. Offer praise for progress. If you feel a need to learn more about BDD, the books and organizations listed in the Resources section may be helpful.

Resources

Body Dysmorphic Disorder and Body Image Dissatisfaction

Berry, Carmen. 1996. *Coming Home to Your Body: 365 Simple Ways to Nourish Yourself Inside and Out*. Berkeley, Calif.: Pagemill Press.

Cash, Thomas F. 1997. *The Body Image Workbook: An 8-Step Program for Learning to Like Your Looks*. Oakland, Calif.: New Harbinger Publications.

Hillman, Carolynn. 1996. *Love Your Looks: How to Stop Criticizing and Start Appreciating Your Appearance*. New York: Fireside.

Johnston, Joni E. 1994. *Appearance Obsession: Learning to Love the Way You Look*. Deerfield Beach, Fla.: Health Communications.

Luciano, Lynne. 2001. *Looking Good: Male Body Image in Modern America*. New York: Hill and Wang.

McBryde, Linda. 1999. *The Mass Market Woman: Defining Yourself as a Person in a World That Defines You by Your Appearance*. Eagle River, Alaska: Crowded Hour Press.

Phillips, Katharine A. 1996. *The Broken Mirror: Understanding and Treating Body Dysmorphic Disorder*. New York: Oxford University Press.

Phillips, Katherine, Barbara Van Noppen, and Leslie Shapiro. 1997. *Learning to Live with BDD*. Milford, Conn.: Obsessive Compulsive Foundation. (A booklet that is especially helpful for family members.)

Pope, Harrison G., Katharine A. Phillips, and Roberto Olivardia. 2000. *The Adonis Complex: The Secret Crisis of Male Body Obsession*. New York: Free Press.

Thompson, Kevin J., Leslie J. Heinberg, Madeline Altabe, and Stacey Tantleff-Dunn. 1999. *Exacting Beauty: Theory, Assessment, and Treatment of Body Image Disturbance.* Washington, D.C.: American Psychological Association.

Obsessive-Compulsive Disorder and Trichotillomania

Baer, Lee. 2000. *Getting Control: Overcoming Your Obsessions and Compulsions. Rev. ed.* New York: Plume.

————. 2001. *The Imp of the Mind: Exploring the Silent Epidemic of Obsessive Bad Thoughts.* New York: E. P. Dutton.

Ciarrocchi, Joseph W. 1995. *The Doubting Disease: Help for Scrupulosity and Religious Compulsions.* Mahwah, N.J.: Paulist Press.

Foa, Edna B., and Reid Wilson. 1991. *Stop Obsessing! How to Overcome Your Obsessions and Compulsions.* New York: Bantam Books.

Hyman, Bruce M., and Cherry Pedrick. 1999. *The OCD Workbook: Your Guide to Breaking Free from Obsessive-Compulsive Disorder.* Oakland, Calif.: New Harbinger Publications.

Keuthen, Nancy J., Dan J. Stein, and Gary A. Christenson. 2001. *Help for Hair Pullers.* Oakland, Calif.: New Harbinger Publications.

Osborn, Ian. 1998. *Tormenting Thoughts and Secret Rituals: The Hidden Epidemic of Obsessive-Compulsive Disorder.* New York: Pantheon Books.

Penzel, Fred. 2000. *Obsessive-Compulsive Disorders: A Complete Guide to Getting Well and Staying Well.* New York: Oxford University Press.

Stein, D., Gary Christenson, and Eric Hollander, eds. 1999. *Trichotillomania.* Washington, D.C.: American Psychiatric Press.

Steketee, Gail S. 1999. *Overcoming Obsessive-Compulsive Disorder: A Behavioral and Cognitive Client Manual.* Oakland, Calif.: New Harbinger Publications.

————. 1999. *Overcoming Obsessive-Compulsive Disorder: A Behavioral and Cognitive Protocol for the Treatment of OCD: Therapist Protocol.* Oakland, Calif.: New Harbinger Publications.

Steketee, Gail, and Kerin White. 1990. *When Once Is Not Enough: Help for Obsessive Compulsives.* Oakland, Calif.: New Harbinger Publications.

Schwartz, Jeffrey, and Beverly Beyette. 1996. *Brain Lock: Free Yourself from Obsessive-Compulsive Behavior.* New York: ReganBooks.

Habit Change

Azrin, Nathan, and Gregory Nunn. 1977. *Habit Control in a Day.* New York: Simon and Schuster.

Claiborn, James, and Cherry Pedrick. 2000. *The Habit Change Workbook: How to Break Bad Habits and Form Good Ones.* Oakland, Calif.: New Harbinger Publications.

Prochaska, James O., John C. Norcross, and Carlo C. DiClemente. 1995. *Changing For Good: A Revolutionary Six-Stage Program for Overcoming Bad Habits and Moving Your Life Positively Forward.* New York: Avon.

Social Anxiety and Self-Esteem

Antony, Martin M., and Richard P. Swinson. 2000. *The Shyness & Social Anxiety Workbook: Proven Techniques for Overcoming Your Fears.* Oakland, Calif.: New Harbinger Publications.

Burns, David D. 1993. *Ten Days to Self-Esteem.* New York: Quill.

Markway, Barbara G., Cheryl N. Carmin, C. Alec Pollard, and Teresa Flynn. 1992. *Dying of Embarassment: Help for Social Anxiety and Phobia.* Oakland, Calif.: New Harbinger Publications.

Markway, Barbara G., and Gregory P. Markway. 2001. *Painfully Shy: How to Overcome Social Anxiety and Reclaim Your Life.* New York: St. Martin's Press.

McKay, Matthew, Patrick Fanning, Carole Honeychurch, and Catharine Sutker. 1999. *The Self-Esteem Companion.* Oakland, Calif.: New Harbinger Publications.

McKay, Matthew, and Patrick Fanning. 2000. *Self-Esteem: A Proven Program of Cognitive Techniques for Assessing, Improving, and Maintaining Your Self-Esteem.* Oakland, Calif.: New Harbinger Publications.

Schneier, Franklin, and Lawrence Welkowitz. 1996. *The Hidden Face of Shyness: Understanding and Overcoming Social Anxiety.* New York: Avon Books.

Stein, Murray B., and John R. Walker. 2001. *Triumph Over Shyness: Conquering Shyness and Social Anxiety.* New York: McGraw-Hill.

Anxiety, Depression, and Relaxation

Burns, David D. 1990. *The Feeling Good Handbook.* New York: Plume.

Bourne, Edmund J. 2000. *The Anxiety and Phobia Workbook.* Oakland, Calif.: New Harbinger Publications.

Copeland, Mary Ellen. 1992. *The Depression Workbook: A Guide to Living with Depression and Manic Depression.* Oakland, Calif.: New Harbinger Publications.

———. 1994. *Living with Depression and Manic Depression.* Oakland, Calif.: New Harbinger Publications.

———. 1998. *The Worry Control Workbook.* Oakland, Calif.: New Harbinger Publications.

Davis, Martha, Elizabeth Robbins Eshelman, and Matthew McKay. 2000. *The Relaxation and Stress Reduction Workbook. 5th ed.* Oakland, Calif.: New Harbinger Publications.

Ellis, Albert. 2001. *Feeling Better, Getting Better, Staying Better: Profound Self-Help Therapy for Your Emotions.* San Luis Obispo, Calif.: Impact.

Langer, Ellen J. 1990. *Mindfulness.* Cambridge, Mass.: Perseus Publishing.

McKay, Matthew, and Patrick Fanning. 1997. *The Daily Relaxer.* Oakland, Calif.: New Harbinger Publications.

Dr. James Claiborn's Recommendations

Kabat-Zinn, Jon. 1994. *Wherever You Go, There You Are: Mindfulness Meditation in Everyday Life.* New York: Hyperion.

———. 1990. *Full Catastrophe Living: Using the Wisdom of Your Body and Mind to Face Stress, Pain, and Illness.* New York: Dell.

Cherry Pedrick's Recommendations

Hart, Archibald D. 1999. *The Anxiety Cure: You Can Find Emotional Tranquility and Wholeness.* Nashville, Tenn.: Word Publishing. (Relaxation tapes are also available.)

McGee, Robert S. 1998. *The Search for Significance.* Nashville, Tenn.: W Publishing Group.

Organizations of Interest

American Foundation for Suicide Prevention, 120 Wall Street, Twenty-second Floor, New York, NY 10005. (212) 363-3500. Internet: http://www.afsp.org

Anorexia Nervosa and Related Eating Disorders., P.O. Box 5102, Eugene, OR 97405. (541) 344-1144. Internet: http://www.anred.com

Anxiety Disorders Association of America, Dept. A, 6000 Executive Blvd., Suite 513, Rockville, MD 20852. (301) 231-9350. Internet: http://www.adaa.org

Association for the Advancement of Behavior Therapy, 305 Seventh Avenue, New York, NY 10001-6008. (212) 647-1890. Internet: http://server.psych.vt.edu/aabt/

Body Dysmorphic Disorder and Body Image Program, Butler Hospital, 345 Blackstone Blvd., Providence, RI 02906. Internet: http://www.butler.org/bdd/

National Alliance for the Mentally Ill, 200 N. Glebe Rd., Suite 1015, Arlington, VA 22203-3754. (800) 950-NAMI (800-950-6264)

National Anxiety Foundation, 3135 Custer Drive, Lexington, KY 40517-4001. (606) 272-7166. Internet: http://lexington-on-line.com/naf.ocd.2.html

National Association of Anorexia Nervosa and Associated Disorders, Box 7, Highland Park, IL 60035. (847) 831-3438. Internet: http://www.healthtouch.com

National Depressive and Manic-Depressive Association, 730 North Franklin, Suite 501, Chicago, IL 60610. (800) 82N-DMDA (800-826-3236)

National Institute of Mental Health, 9000 Rockville Pike, Building 10. Room 30-41, Bethesda, MD 20892. (301) 496-3421. Information services: panic and other anxiety disorders: (800) 647-2642; depression: (800) 421-4211

Obsessive-Compulsive Foundation., P.O. Box 70, Milford, CT 06460-0070. (203) 878-5669. Internet: http://www.ocfoundation.org

The President's Council on Physical Fitness and Sports, 400 Sixteenth Avenue NW, Washington, DC 20036

Trichotillomania Learning Center, 303 Potrero, Suite 51, Santa Cruz, CA 95060. (831) 457-1004. Internet: http://www.trich.org/

References

American Psychiatric Association. 1987. *Diagnostic and Statistical Manual of Mental Disorders (DSM-III-R)*. 3rd ed. Revised. Washington, D.C.: American Psychiatric Association.

————. 2000. *Diagnostic and Statistical Manual of Mental Disorders, (DSM-IV-TR)*. 4th ed. Text revision. Washington, D.C.: American Psychiatric Association.

Azrin, Nathan, and Gregory Nunn. 1977. *Habit Control in a Day*. New York: Simon and Schuster.

Beck, Judith S. 1995. *Cognitive Therapy: Basics and Beyond*. New York: Guilford Press.

Benson, Herbert, and Eileen M. Stuart. 1993. *The Wellness Book: The Comprehensive Guide to Maintaining Health and Treating Stress-Related Illness*. New York: Fireside.

Burns, David D. 1993. *The Feeling Good Handbook*. New York: Plume.

Cash, Thomas F. 1997. *The Body Image Workbook: An 8-Step Program for Learning to Like Your Looks*. Oakland, Calif.: New Harbinger Publications.

Hart, Archibald D. 1999. *The Anxiety Cure: You Can Find Emotional Tranquility and Wholeness*. Nashville, Tenn.: Word Publishing.

Jolanta, J. Rabe-Jablonska, and M. Sobow Tomasz. 2000. The links between body dysmorphic disorder and eating disorders. *European Psychiatry* 15(5):302–330.

Kabat-Zinn Jon. 1994. *Wherever You Go, There You Are: Mindfulness Meditation in Everyday Life*. New York: Hyperion.

Langer, Ellen J. 1990. *Mindfulness*. Cambridge, Mass.: Perseus Publishing.

Linehan, Marsha M. 1993. *Skills Training Manual for Treating Borderline Personality Disorder*. New York: Guilford Press.

Luciano, Lynne. 2001. *Looking Good: Male Image in Modern America*. New York: Hill and Wang.

Marlatt, G. Alan. 1985. Relapse prevention: Theoretical rationale and overview of the model. In *Relapse Prevention*, edited by G. Alan Marlatt and Judith R. Gordon. New York: Guilford Press.

Miltenberger, R. G., W. R. Fuqua, and D. W. Woods. 1998. Applying behavior analysis to clinical problems: Review and analysis of habit reversal. *Journal of Applied Behavior Analysis* 31:447–469.

Phillips, Katharine A. 1996. *The Broken Mirror: Understanding and Treating Body Dysmorphic Disorder*. New York: Oxford University Press.

———. 1999. Body dysmorphic disorder and depression: Theoretical considerations and treatment strategies. *Psychiatric Quarterly* 4:313–331.

Phillips, Katharine A., Raymond G. Dufrense, Caroline S. Wilkel, and Carmela C. Vittorio. 2000. Rate of body dysmorphic disorder in dermatology patients. *Journal of the American Academy of Dermatology* 42:436–441.

Phillips, Katharine A., Eric Hollander, Steven Rasmussen, Bonnie Aronowitz, Concetta DeCaria, and Wayne Goodman. 1997. A severity rating scale for body dysmorphic disorder: Development, reliability, and validity of a modified version of the Yale-Brown Obsessive Compulsive Scale. *Psychopharmacology Bulletin* 33:17–22.

Phillips, Katharine A., and Susan L. McElroy. 2000. Personality disorders and traits in patients with body dysmorphic disorder. *Comprehensive Psychiatry* 41:229–236.

Pope, Harrison G., Katharine A. Phillips, and Roberto Olivardia. 2000. *The Adonis Complex: The Secret Crisis of Male Body Obsession*. New York: Free Press.

Prochaska, James O., Carlo C. DiClemente, and John C. Norcross. 1992. In search of how people change: Applications to addictive behaviors. *American Psychologist* 47:1102–1114

Prochaska, James O., John C. Norcross, and Carlo C. DiClemente. 1995. *Changing For Good: A Revolutionary Six Stage Program for Overcoming Bad Habits and Moving Your Life Positively Forward*. New York: Avon.

Schwartz, Jeffrey, and Beverly Beyette. 1996. *Brain Lock: Free Yourself from Obsessive-Compulsive Behaviors*. New York: Regan Books.

Some Other
New Harbinger Titles

Watercooler Wisdom, Item 4364 $14.95

The Juicy Tomato Guide to Ripe Living After 50, Item 4321 $16.95

What's Right With Me, Item 4429 $16.95

The Balanced Mom, Item 4534 $14.95

Women Who Worry Too Much, Item 4127 $13.95

In Harm's Way, Item 4003 $14.95

Breastfeeding Made Simple, Item 4046 $16.95

The Well-Ordered Office, Item 3856 $13.95

Talk to Me, Item 3317 $12.95

Romantic Intelligence, Item 3309 $15.95

Transformational Divorce, Item 3414 $13.95

The Rape Recovery Handbook, Item 3376 $15.95

Eating Mindfully, Item 3503 $13.95

Sex Talk, Item 2868 $12.95

Everyday Adventures for the Soul, Item 2981 $11.95

A Woman's Addiction Workbook, Item 2973 $19.95

The Daughter-In-Law's Survival Guide, Item 2817 $12.95

PMDD, Item 2833 $13.95

The Vulvodynia Survival Guide, Item 2914 $16.95

Love Tune-Ups, Item 2744 $10.95

Brave New You, Item 2590 $13.95

The Woman's Book of Sleep, Item 2493 $14.95

Pregnancy Stories, Item 2361 $14.95

The Women's Guide to Total Self-Esteem, Item 2418 $14.95

The Conscious Bride, Item 2132 $12.95

Juicy Tomatoes, Item 2175 $14.95

High on Stress, Item 1101 $13.95

Perimenopause, 2nd edition, Item 2345 $17.95

The Infertility Survival Guide, Item 2477 $16.95

Call **toll free, 1-800-748-6273,** or log on to our online bookstore at **www.newharbinger.com** to order. Have your Visa or Mastercard number ready. Or send a check for the titles you want to New Harbinger Publications, Inc., 5674 Shattuck Ave., Oakland, CA 94609. Include $4.50 for the first book and 75¢ for each additional book, to cover shipping and handling. (California residents please include appropriate sales tax.) Allow two to five weeks for delivery.

Prices subject to change without notice.